# Turning Point

## A Pathway out of Alzheimer's

Written by Robert L Ruisi

5/06/2016

*I have been walking on air wondering where to begin the amazing story I have to share. It is my personal story of finding a pathway out of Alzheimer's. I hope that sharing this will help many others suffering from Alzheimer's Disease, Dementia and other memory loss illnesses.*

# Introduction

I am about to share explosive news with you in the hopes that it will help many people who are suffering from Alzheimer's, dementia and any other memory loss illness.

I have Alzheimer's disease. I can't say I don't have it any longer, but I can say I have improved to an amazing level. This is my story.

# Table of Contents

# Chapter 1
# Background

In 1968, I started out as a panhandler on Market Street in San Francisco. Soon after, in 69, I joined the corporate world in New York City. I quickly worked my way up ladder from filing invoices for the bookkeeper, to order processing, and then onto sales. I started out as clerical help and before long I was promoted to sales. I was a natural at it. It was almost as if I could wave a magic wand, and there would appear another order and a new account. The company was pleased with the clients I brought in, which included Sears.

Being a detail-oriented person, I'd carefully plan out every action on each client account and determine what I would sell to them. I set up my weekly, monthly and long- term goals. I made sure that each goal was realistic and reachable. My only competition was myself, always pushing to beat the numbers I had achieved the previous week.

My father passed away when I was quite young. I watched as he faded away due to cancer and observed how my mother responded to the moment. Before passing, my father gave me a piece of advice: *keep business small* and you'll always make money. When my father died, it affected every aspect of my life. I guess you could say that I lost my sense of direction and my guide. I took the guilty sons detour for a brief moment in time. Later, his advice would help me chose a small business – I wanted to be close to home and enjoy my family before the same thing happened to me.

I was successful at what I did, but I wanted more. I needed something for myself, including the ability to use my own unique expression and creativity. Like everyone in America, I wanted to start my own business someday. So, I set up a goal and started working in that direction. Finally, I began to experiment with a small business, which I treated like a toy. When one thing did not work out, I tried another idea until it did.

I understood so called 'big business' but never wanted it for myself. I chose to engage in a small business for two reasons. I did not want the responsibility of a large business or the corporate politics that would necessarily accompany it. I had seen that scenario all too often. My father and his two partners built a large size corporation for their day, but that business approach was not for me. I liked working shoulder-to-shoulder and eye-to-eye with people. I felt it was a more honest lifestyle, plus I enjoyed the freedom of expression. I could "move on a dime" and that was very strategic for my success.

After spending some years playing my personal "game of chess," I developed a business that was as easy as one, two, three. It had taken me a long time to accomplish this goal because I had been looking for the perfect option. The business had to be simple and easy to control, almost running itself. I established a small import company that ran like clockwork, which was perfect for my needs—not that I ever wanted all that much.

I married at eighteen to a woman who was a year younger than me. We were a couple of kids really, just starting out, and we ended up having three wonderful girls. As kids do, they grew up and started their own families.

Over the years, my wife and I grew in different ways and directions – worlds apart – as many couples do. She enjoyed the benefits of my accomplishments, loved to go out to eat and spent life casually; her responsibilities were directed toward family affairs. By the time this story starts, my responsibilities were all about the business. We ultimately divorced after my diagnoses, too hot in the kitchen I guess, but it was surely for the best and I do wish her luck.

# Chapter 2
# Beginning

Over a two-year period, I began to experience some stomach issues that caused a slight discomfort in my abdomen. At the time, I did not think much of these occurrences. Now, as I look back, I can understand what was going on. The stomach issues came in a cycle, and with each cycle the discomfort increased. Additionally, loose bowel movements added to the unpleasantness. *(What a note to start on!)*

Fast forward to 2006. I was heading to upstate New York for an appointment and left home around 3:00 a.m. The sun was rising as I drove, and was shining its morning light on the trees along the road side. with deep appreciation, I took in all the beauty I was seeing.

The slight abdominal discomfort was present when I started the trip, but I didn't feel it was serious enough to be concerned about. I kept thinking it would pass and tried to make myself as comfortable as possible. I focused my attention on the drive, admiring the hilltops along the way.

At this point, it is important to mention that my birth mother had recently been diagnosed with Alzheimer's disease. It was notably odd how it was first discovered. She had been writing notes to herself for a few years, and everyone just kidded her about it. One day, while she was visiting my younger half-brother Gerry, she was not as argumentative as usual. He was alarmed and said, "Something is wrong with mom!"

I thought nothing of it, and neither did my two half-sisters. "Gerry is just overreacting," we said. He insisted that his mother see a doctor and, sure enough, he was right. So, that's why she was keeping all those notes, I thought, and I went about my business.

The appointment in New York was with a client named Keith, who I'd always felt was a good businessman. I thought highly of him and his opinions. Keith ran a small chain of discount stores in the New England area, about 35 in all, and was known to be honest in his dealings—as rare as that may seem these days. The two of us shared a lot in common, as we were both self-made businessmen with down-to-earth personalities.

I had gone through my usual show and tell - at least that was what I called it. Keith asked all of the usual questions – how much, when and where? As always, I had the answers ready. He placed his orders, which included a couple of container loads from China plus some 'immediate delivery goods' closeouts. I was very thankful for the business he gave me and packed up my sample cases. I was ready to head off to my next appointment on the following day.

As I packed the car, my stomach was still causing me a great deal of discomfort. Driving over long distances, one is always concerned about that type of problem, and the necessary pit stops! I didn't think too much of it. I got into the car, went to fill it up with gas, and grabbed a *diet soda*. I'd had a good morning's sale with Keith, which totaled about forty-eight thousand dollars' worth of merchandise. It wasn't a bad way to start my trip.

I had a long drive ahead of me and after arriving at the mini-mart/gas station, I first went to get a *diet soda*. I then filled up the gas tank for the long trip that was ahead of. Afterwards, I went inside the mini-mart to buy a pack of cigarettes. I should mention here that *diet soda* is not a friend to your brain. I did not know it at the time and have long since cut it near out of my life along. I also stopped smoking *cigarettes*, which are also not good for your brain or your lungs.

Ready for the journey, I headed toward the interstate highway. With my stomach still causing me pain, I wiggled around to get comfortable in my seat, and continued to ignore the pangs all the way to Maryland. I had no idea what was causing it. It was consistent and uncomfortable, and I chose to focus on the outside view as a distraction.

When I arrived in Maryland, I got a room for the night. I ate a simple dinner and drank a soda before heading off to bed. I wanted to make an early night of it and be fresh for my early appointment the next day. Throughout the night my stomach bothered me.

When I woke the next morning, my stomach was still aching but not as bad. I got ready for my appointment and paid the hotel bill. I went for a light and simple breakfast, ordering an egg and cheese sandwich. I also had my *diet soda*, which never left my side. After finishing, I headed off to my appointment. I sat in the car waiting for the buyer, Nels, to arrive.

Nels is an owner of a distribution company, Rainbow Sales, specializing in non-foods for supermarkets. He and I are around the same age, and have a lot in common. Both of us were self-made businessmen who grew up in the 60s. Nels ran his business with a great deal of care and like myself was very detail orientated. He had to be a detail person, as the supermarket business is a tough trade to be in. I always looked forward to seeing Nels and thought of him as a good friend.

I leaned back in my car and had a smoke while preparing my paperwork and samples. The cell phone rang, and it was my wife checking in to find out my progress. I was always a bit hidden about my progress. I felt it was bad luck to count my chickens before they hatched.

Nels pulled up and we went inside the building and I did my usual show and tell. He picked out plenty of goods, asking all of the usual questions, to which I gave answers. I always provided him with detailed information.

At the end of our meeting, Nels told me, "I'll place the order in a few days."

"Hey, thanks, Nels," I replied, packing up my samples and paperwork.

I loaded my car and headed off to see another account in the area. That day I saw 3 more accounts including Star Imports, Your Wholesale, and another before heading back to my home office. On the way, I stopped for a *diet soda* and gas. I was pleased with myself. I had a home run at each appointment I thought. Some accounts were smaller than others but it all added up.

All the way back my stomach was bothering me. I did not know why, nor did I pay it much attention. After all, I was a busy businessman. *I have to say after looking back this was a signal that I should have paid closer attention to!*

I was feeling tired and as my stomach issues grew it was becoming more difficult to complete my normal daily routines. Considering the way I worked, it was not surprising that I would wear down from time to time. I did, and would, wear out every so many years, but this was something different.

During one of my business trips I purchased property in upstate New York. It was a small house, with 2 rental units. It had one tenant already occupying the lower portion of the house, and with a little tender loving care the upper unit would be ready to rent out as well. Over a one year period I had the house fixed, rented out, and back on the market for sale. This was my first real estate deal and if successful I had planned on moving a healthy portion of the business into real estate with the hope of easing my life. I was getting older and was thinking about retirement.

Sure enough the house sold in no time to an investor from the UK. I did extremely well for my first time trying out this sort of venture. I started planning the next investment. I had my eye on 24 units plus a building. A young man was handling a lot of the work based on a rental deal for him. It was a sound plan, and he was an honest hard working young man. The only slight issue was at the time I was in New Jersey, and this deal was in upstate New York. It not be an easy trip, even though many times I had driven further.

Keep in mind that during this time I was feeling tired and it whatever was wrong was getting worse. Traveling was becoming a concern and something else was starting to happen. I was getting lost or what I would call taking the long way home! This was a problem. I was getting slightly lost going to places I traveled all the time. Keep in mind I would drive out from New Jersey all the way to Branson, MO or as far south as Miami, FL, and now I was getting lost coming back from Philadelphia, Baltimore, and even Kearney, New Jersey. There was clearly something going on.

Starting from this point, every choice I made was based upon what was happening. It was not the way to run a business, and none of the choices I made were to my advantage. Actually, every choice I made from that point on failed and ultimately cost me the business in the end. I was not thinking clearly. I had lost my mathematical skills. I was getting lost and forgetting things. I was also losing weight rapidly. One could easily say I was making decisions out of desperation, but was it in desperation or was I just out of it? I'm not sure that I even know, as I look back at the process.

There are a few key items I wish to mention in closing this chapter. My diet was not made up of healthy choices. I drank diet coke like most drink water. I looked it up online and there is actually a diet coke addiction! Can you believe tit is easy to become addicted to drinking diet coke? I sometimes wonder about humans, and their choices. Diet Coke was my only intake of fluids, and that was not a brain healthy choice. Also, I had smoked most of my life, which is another unhealthy brain choice. Lastly, my sleep patterns where not working in my favor. I would sleep for just a couple of hours daily and did that for most of my career. Four hours per night was common place, and once again it was not a healthy brain choice.

# Chapter 3
# Doctors

Normally I could pick myself up when things were down. I had been in tight situations before as a businessman, but this time I simply did not have the strength. I was weakened by whatever was going on with my body. I lost the business and filed personal bankruptcy. It was now 2010.

My weight went from 196 down to 122 pounds. I was flat broke and in need of a doctors' help to find out what was wrong. I went to see Doctor Angelo T Scotti of Little Silver, New Jersey. Because of my financial condition Dr Scotti recommended that I should to sign up for charity care with Parker House in Red Bank New Jersey (clearly this is before the ACA act. No one knows what was lost by that bill.) I had to sign up there at Parker House and at Riverview Hospital, also in Red Bank. Lucky for me charity care accepted me into their program, which meant free doctors' visits.

Parker House Clinic employed a nice group of doctors, nurses, and other support staff members. I remember sitting there on my first visit and looking at the wall of photos. It contained various donors; some I knew, some I knew of, and then some I knew not at all. There at Parker House Clinic my age did not work in my favor, and rather than listening to the patient they drew their own conclusions without using medical expertise. They assumed age limited all possibilities of finding a solution.

Parker House Clinic ran test after test with preset and preconceived notions. They gave me blood tests and those for urine and stool. They took my blood pressure each time I went and checked my heart rate. "Everything is good," they would say. "We can't find anything wrong with you." They assigned a psychologist for me to meet with. She was another nice gal but did not listen and with preconceived beliefs said, "You're depressed." She sent me to CPC, which was also in Red Bank. I could not believe what I was hearing. I told them I was not depressed. I was not happy about my situation, but who would be happy considering what I was going through and experiencing? Depressed was not my way of handling anything. I was pissed offed that I was not standing up and doing what I had done all of my life. Hey, you fall off you horse you get back up on the darn thing and ride!

CPC turned out to be the best thing that had happened in a long time. I set up the appointment, and it was with Susan Grant MD. I remember sitting in the waiting room wondering where is this going to lead? Will I be heard or just pushed into a never-ending system? I brought with me a "sequence of events" chart that I had made for Parker House Clinic. I met with Susan, showed her my chart, and told her how I felt. It took maybe 5 minutes and she said, "You have to see a neurologist right-a-way" She wrote a note for the hospital, everything had to go through them (charity care rules). The hospital immediately set me up with Doctor Richard Rhee in Neptune New Jersey.

Once at Dr. Rhee's office he gave me the written test. I was drawing clocks, images, memorizing information, and doing some mathematics. I was not showing good signs. Something was wrong, and he sent me for more tests. Each test was to identify what was wrong and verify if I did, or did not, have Alzheimer's. First they did a test to verify I had the markers for Alzheimer's checking the genes. It was not a hard test to go through, and yes, the tests came back positive. I did have the markers for the disease.

Dr. Rhee also sent me for an MRI. That was not so much fun, and noisy is not even the word I would use to describe it! They give you ear plugs. My goodness, as I laid there unable to move until prompted, pops, whistles, and pounding sounds were continual. The ear plugs did not seem to have any effect and the sounds were not being muffled!

There is an specific process you go through with most of these tests, and I will write about them later.

As each of the test results were coming back in, it was quickly becoming clear I had Alzheimer's disease. Because of my age it was called early-onset Alzheimer's. It was not the most common of the Alzheimer's disease group, but clearly by the name not unheard of either. There are 3 types of Alzheimer's diseases including early-onset, late-onset, and familial.

Early-onset Alzheimer's happens to people who are under the age of 65. They can even be as young as 30, but more commonly the symptoms start to show signs in the 40's or 50's. Mine showed up in my 50's as did my birth mother's. Because it is rare, it is often over-looked by doctors at first. Less than 10% of all people with Alzheimer's have early-onset. People that do have it tend to have more of the brain changes that are linked with Alzheimer's. The early-onset form also appears to be linked with a defect in a specific part of a person's DNA: chromosome 14.  A form of muscle twitching and spasm, called myoclonus, is also more common in early-onset Alzheimer's.

Late-onset Alzheimer's is the most common form of the disease, which happens to people age 65 and older. It may or may not run in families. So far, researchers haven't found a particular gene that causes it. No one knows for sure why some people get it and others don't.

Familial Alzheimer's disease (FAD), is a form of Alzheimer's disease that doctors know for certain is linked to genes. In families that are affected, members of at least two generations have had the disease. FAD makes up less than 1% of all cases of Alzheimer's. People who have it start showing signs very early, often in their 40s.

The mother of a friend of mine was suffering with Alzheimer's disease and was doing well in a study group with Dr. Joel Ross MD. I was given his telephone number and promptly gave his office a call. They scheduled an appointment to evaluate me for the next program he was starting. He gave me written tests and some open question and answers, a blood workup, and sent me to get a PET scan.

Physicians that are diagnosing dementia or Alzheimer's can study the structure of the patient's brain by CT or MRI to see if there are any growths, abnormalities, or general shrinkage (as noted in cases of Alzheimer's). Studies of brain function, using a PET scan and a special form of MRI can more definitively confirm the diagnosis of various types of dementia and increase the precision of the diagnosis up to 90%. A PET scan administered and reviewed by experts does deliver the most accurate and suggestive results diagnosing dementia. The most precise form of PET scanning for types of dementia is called Stereotactic Surface Projection, which involves an advanced statistical analysis of the data.

The precision using the PET scan tests is 90% with regards to Alzheimer's and frontotemporal dementia types. Experts agree that scans increased the confidence in diagnosing dementia types and made them question and often change their original diagnosis in 42% of cases. They stated that early and accurate diagnosing of dementia is critical to avoid misdiagnosis and mistreatment. The results of this study show that PET scanning is highly predictive of the patient's clinical course and essential to properly diagnosing dementia. I had the PET scan, and can say this is a very effective tool in diagnosing.

The PET scan and the MRI tests that I had gone through showed; brain shrinkage, clogged blood vessels in the brain, and plaque. I have Alzheimer's. I chose not to be in Dr. Ross's study group. Being a lab rat was not my idea of fun and there were possible risks. Nope, it was not for me! Dr. Richard Rhee wrote the subscription for Donepezil, 10 MG per day, and Later increased it to 20 MG, plus he added Namenda 10 MG and later increased that. I was at the maximum strength I could take!

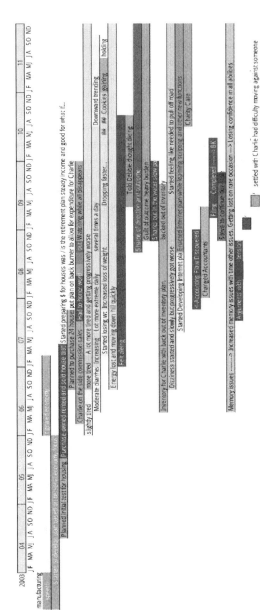

# Chapter 4
# Turning Point

I was doing everything I could to be active. Between playing with my grandchildren and making friends on Facebook, I was involved and trying to continue to function normally. I was being normal with whatever the new normal was!

I was fully engaged on Facebook, and I would make online friends and communicate with everyone. Often I was sharing and debating opinions about this that or the other thing, saying just enough to keep the pot stirred lightly. I was also helping other writers online by sharing their amazon ads, which displayed their work. My mind was active. There is an old saying that comes to mind, "An active mind cannot exist in an inactive body." And both body and mind were active! I was not at all shy about telling people I had Alzheimer's. In fact, I felt I needed a backup system just in case I slipped up.

Friends online were sharing information pertaining to Alzheimer's disease and not so well-known natural remedies. I would read the material and research the information. My daughter was doing the same thing, and there was tons of information being shared with us. The online community of friends I had built up over time was so very helpful. We investigated the natural remedies being suggested and little by little I would add one to my daily intake. Of course we shared whatever I was adding with my doctors just to be sure nothing would interfere with the meds that I was on.

My oldest daughter and I had been researching Alzheimer's disease for a period of time. Particularly, I studied the causes of the disease, including some of the offbeat causes which are still in debate by those who are invested in receiving funding for the ongoing research! Alzheimer's in most, if not all, cases is genetic and people have the markers in their genes for the disease. There are a lot of the triggers activating the disease. Some triggers lay in the environment and the foods we consume while others have to do with lifestyle. Depression is known for bringing on dementia and Alzheimer's disease.

I have to say the beginning of my turning point started with the addition of coconut oil. I was taking coconut oil with Omega 3,6,9, D3, and E along with B12. But when I added the coconut oil there was a difference. I seemed to be able to communicate a bit better, and when I was out of coconut oil for just a few days I became more withdrawn. It was a clear help to me.

One day 3 different Facebook users, plus my daughter, all told me about a news story released by Huffington Post and sent me links to the story line. I was reading the story and could not believe it, but then all these people alerted me so it must have meaning! As I read about Paul Stamets of Fungi.net and his Lion's Mane mushroom, I quickly checked Paul's reputation, and it is impeccable. As I looked at this new information, and I saw it as some sort of sign, I quickly decided to give this stuff a try. I was trying everything else with some success, so why not this? I found a couple of places online that were selling Lion's Mane, and one of the places was carrying Paul Stamets brand. I purchased it. and within a few days I started taking the suggested dosage based upon my weight at the time. I was by that time up to 183 because my daughter is a good cook. What can I say?

I can't say enough good things about Lion's Mane. Within 30 days after I started taking Lion's Mane I started to notice something happening. After two months I knew what I was noticing, and it was big, really big. Each month thereafter I improved more, and I could not believe what was going on, I mean, I was thrown for one heck of a loop.

Susan Grant MD, my psychiatrist, was noticing the changes too. I should add she had taken me off the meds that she was subscribing over the course of several months. But this visit was different she noticed how much I had improved and felt I needed to see my neurologist for evaluation. You have to understand you just don't get better with Alzheimer's. At least it has not happened before, and yet I clearly was improving.

I was feeling mighty good and eagerly set up the appointment to see Dr. Richard Rhee. Sitting in his office a lot of thoughts were flying. I knew how I was feeling, and I knew Susan noticed the difference, but how would that translate with Dr. Rhee, I wondered. Richard and I spoke briefly once I arrived in his office. He was surprised that my oldest daughter did not come. He then gave me the standard "let's see how much worse you are doing test" When I was done, Dr. Rhee's eyes lit up mouth dropped and said "You've improved!"

Mind you, this just does not happen, not with Alzheimer's. He took me off Namenda and continued the scripts for Donepezil. We scheduled the next appointment and there I know the donepezil will be reduced if not removed all together. I would not say I am 100% better, but I will say I am getting darn close to it. Every month I am noting more improvement, every month!

*My personal belief is it is a combination that has helped me recover. Daily exercise (both mental and physical), a stress free environment, vitamins, supplements, and lots of laughter is what has improved my health.*

Just think for a moment about the choices I could have made during this process. I could have said "no, I am not going to try something else…" I could have chosen not to even looked at the information! **Turning point**, just when the *road forks* which way do you turn?

# Chapter 5
# Vitamins

# My Daily Regimen of Vitamins

| | | | |
|---|---|---|---|
| B12 | 1000 mg | 1 | morning |
| D3 | 1000 iu | 1 | morning |
| Vitamin E complex | 400 iu | 1 | morning |
| C | 500 mg | 1 | morning |

## B12

As I was getting worse, I was in the care of my oldest daughter. She suggested after reading various online information I start taking some of the above mentioned vitamins; B12, D3 and E. Later I added C which was more to resist colds than any other reason. Each of these is helpful for your brain and shown to have results.

## Facts why your body needs B12

Your body relies on vitamin B12 for energy production. It's a key part of the metabolic process that converts carbohydrates and fats into energy — this is why it's often called the "energy vitamin."

B12 is one of the building blocks your body uses to produce DNA. It's vital for healthy cell growth and repair. Proper levels of B12 keep your immune system functioning optimally, regulate mood and sleep cycles and lessen the harmful effects of the toxic stress hormone homocysteine.

New research is showing that B12's most vital function of all may be protecting your brain and entire nervous system. It does this by keeping your nerves communicating in an optimal manner.

## Advantages for the Brain

Vitamin B12 plays a particularly critical role in a properly functioning human brain as well as the nervous system. B12 is critical and important; first, it is important to understand that B12 plays a role in the metabolism of every cell of your body. Secondly, it also plays a role in DNA synthesis and is of great importance for pregnant women and nursing mothers. Yet, in recent years, it is B12's role in brain aging and brain health that has received a great deal of attention.

## Healthy Aging Brain

Due to the fact that B12 works to keep the brain healthy, this powerful vitamin is being studied as a way of combating *brain shrinkage* in the elderly. Maintaining proper B12 levels in the body is a way to keep one's brain healthy, as it may fight off everything from *memory loss* problems to depression.

A variety of studies have currently strongly indicated that a B12 deficiency can lead to *brain shrinkage* and numerous other brain and nervous system related problems. This fact means that B12 consumption in the elderly is of great importance. Those looking to fight off *cognitive decline* in all its forms will be well served by eating B12 rich foods and taking a high quality B vitamin supplement of some kind.

The best food sources of Vitamin B12 include: eggs, milk, cheese, milk products, meat, fish, shellfish and poultry. Some soy and rice beverages as well as soy based meat substitutes are fortified with vitamin B12. To see if a product contains vitamin B12 check the Nutrition Facts on the food label.

# D3

## Vitamin D and the adult and aging brain

Recent epidemiological studies state that too-low levels of vitamin D apparently raise peoples' danger of fatal stroke, dementia, and multiple sclerosis (MS). In recent research by, Thomas Wang of Harvard Medical School in Boston followed 1,739 people (average age 59) for 5 years. Those with low vitamin D levels had about a 60 percent higher risk of a cardiovascular event such as heart attack or stroke than did those having higher levels of the nutrient, even after accounting for other well-known cardiovascular risk factors for example diabetes, high cholesterol, and high blood pressure. The risk for heart attack, heart failure, or stroke was double in people with both high blood pressure and vitamin D deficiency.

Investigators at the University of Heidelberg in Germany reported similar results. Of 3,316 people referred for evaluation of their heart arteries, those with low levels of vitamin D were more likely to have a fatal stroke in the next seven years (the median follow-up period), even after accounting for other cardiovascular risk factors. These authors noted that vitamin D thins the blood and seems to protect neurons in animal studies; the researchers' findings suggested that people who have had strokes, or are at high risk for stroke, should take vitamin D supplements. Findings from a number of studies in which researchers induced strokes in animals also support the idea that a certain level of vitamin D can prevent or treat stroke.

The results of these studies are consistent with psychiatric research investigating the cognitive and mental impairment associated with the age-related decline in vitamin D levels referred to as hypovitaminosis D (HVD). At least 40 percent—one study indicated 90 percent—of older adults, including people who live in sunny areas such as Florida, have HVD. Because vitamin D is fat soluble, many elderly people (who often have a higher fat-to-muscle ratio) may retain more of the nutrient in fatty tissue and have less of it available in the blood to maintain proper health. In addition, as we age, our skin becomes less efficient at making vitamin D from the sun.

A recent review of the research on vitamin D deficiency and mental disorders by Paul Cherniack's group at the University of Miami found five studies reporting an association between HVD and dementia, four studies linking it to mood disorders such as depression and bipolar disorder and four studies linking it to schizophrenia. Only two studies to date found no relationship between HVD and mental illness: one study of depression and one study of dementia.

The bulk of the evidence so far suggests that people who have HVD are at greater risk for conditions such as stroke, dementia, and mood disorders than those who do not. What is not clear is whether short-term oral vitamin D supplements would reverse these conditions in people who already have them. Again, more research is needed.

A critical issue in designing future clinical studies is defining the optimal dosage of oral vitamin D. For example, Reinhold Vieth, a prominent vitamin D researcher from the University of Toronto, has argued persuasively that clinical trials should use oral vitamin D doses equal to or higher than 800 IU/day (an International Unit, or IU, is a measurement based on a vitamin's biological effect), since most previous studies reporting clinical benefits of vitamin D for bone health used doses that exceeded this level. Already one trial using supplements to treat people with depression that used only 400 IU/day (the current U.S. recommended daily allowance for adults, also described as 5 micrograms) failed to show any benefit from the treatment.

One of the most active areas of vitamin D research is its potential connection to multiple sclerosis (MS). As is the case with autism, the number of people with MS is higher in northern latitudes. Since vitamin D is produced primarily by exposure to sunlight, and high serum levels of vitamin D have been reported to correlate with a reduced risk of MS, researchers hypothesize that vitamin D may help protect people from the disease.

A recent study conducted by scientists at the University of Oxford and the University of British Columbia is being hailed by many as a major step in proof of this hypothesis because it links the environmental risk factor of low vitamin D levels with a previously known genetic abnormality common to many people with MS. These researchers discovered that if a person has low levels of vitamin D, this gene does not function properly, which sets up vulnerability to environmental triggers suspected in MS. At least two clinical trials are under way to investigate the potential benefits of using vitamin D supplements as a treatment for MS.

We find compelling the scientific evidence from animal studies that vitamin D supports healthy brain function in general throughout life. Vitamin D appears to be a "multi-potent" brain-cell-protective hormone, working through diverse and complex mechanisms including brain calcium regulation, anti-oxidative properties, immune system regulation and enhanced brain cell signaling.

http://www.dana.org/Cerebrum/2009/Vitamin_D_and_th e_Brain__More_Good_News/#sthash.JeCAC5gA.dpuf

*Dr. Mercola writes, Vitamin D has been shown to improve a number of brain disorders, including dementia and its most severe form, Alzheimer's disease, the latter of which now affects an estimated 5.2 million Americans.*

# Vitamin E complex

The following was copied from life-enhancement.com

Vitamin E Keeps Your Brain Razor-Sharp for those with suboptimal levels; it can improve cognitive age by 8-9 years.

By Aaron W. Jensen, Ph.D.

You're committed to better health, right? You've decided that you're going to do your best to eat right, stay in shape, and improve your healthy outlook on life. After all, you've got a lot to live for. You want to live long, live well, and by all means keep your brain sharp - because physical health means nothing without a lively brain. (No matter how powerful a computer's hardware components may be, it's just a big paperweight if the CPU is "fried.")

So you set yourself to the task. At the dinner table, you heap vegetables onto your plate, eat fish, turkey, and chicken rather than red meat, and try to forgo dessert. At lunchtime you eat salads instead of fast food. And at breakfast, you ditch the muffins and doughnuts in favor of fortified, low-glycemic cereals and a colorful selection of fresh fruit. Good for you! You're doing all the right things. Well, maybe not all. A nagging question remains: are you getting all the vitamins, minerals, and other nutrients you need to live life to the fullest and remain mentally acute?

## Most Americans Need More Vitamin E

Nutritional surveys show that most Americans are deficient in some extremely important vitamins and minerals. For example, most of us don't get as much vitamin E from dietary sources as we should, because we don't eat enough vitamin E-rich foods (such as nuts and seeds). Just because you have a good diet doesn't necessarily mean that you're getting all the important nutrients you need in the amounts you need. This is especially true of older people, whose bodies no longer extract certain nutrients from food as efficiently as they once did.

A significant number of adults in the USA - 28% of women and 29% of men - have low serum levels of vitamin E

A national health survey (NHANES III, the National Health and Nutrition Examination Survey) was conducted between 1988 and 1994 to determine the typical nutrient intake of Americans. Investigators at the Centers for Disease Control and Prevention (CDC) analyzed the data, which were collected from 16,300 adults 18 years of age or older, and they concluded that a significant number of adults in the USA - 28% of women and 29% of men -

have low serum levels of vitamin E (even by the low standards of recommended intake applied in the survey).1 Further analysis revealed that 41% of blacks, 28% of Mexican-Americans, and 26% of whites have low vitamin E levels. Clearly, getting sufficient vitamin E is a problem for many of us (see the sidebar).

### Dietary Sources of Vitamin E

Supplementation with vitamin E is advisable for everyone, mainly for the well-established cardiovascular benefits it offers. That doesn't mean, however, that you should overlook good dietary sources of this wonderful vitamin. Although it's almost impossible to have a clinical vitamin E deficiency, many diets are low in this substance; mainly because they contain a lot of processed foods (processing destroys vitamin E). And the diets of some health zealots are very low - sometimes too low - in fat, which can be problematic because most vitamin E comes from fatty foods, such as vegetable oils, nuts, and seeds.

Best Dietary Sources of Vitamin E

| Food Item | Serving Size | Vitamin E Content (mg ATE) |
|---|---|---|
| Assorted fortified cereals | 3/4-1 cup | 20 |
| Sunflower seeds | 1 oz | 14.2 |
| Almonds | 1 oz | 7.4 |
| Sunflower oil | 1 tbsp | 6.9 |
| Canned tomato purée | 1 cup | 6.3 |
| Turnip greens | 1 cup | 4.8 |
| Safflower oil | 1 tbsp | 4.7 |
| Hazelnuts | 1 oz | 4.3 |
| Spinach | 1 cup | 2.8 |
| Peanuts | 1 oz | 2.1 |

Source: USDA Nutrient Database. The abbreviation "mg ATE" stands for "milligrams of alpha-tocopherol equivalents," a way of expressing the biological activity of vitamin E. A more common unit of measure for vitamin E is the international unit (IU).

Our Brains Need Abundant Vitamin E

Vitamin E has received a huge amount of press lately, because it's an important antioxidant - one of those beneficial nutrients that protect our tissues from the destructive effects of free radicals.* An important aspect of vitamin E's role as an antioxidant is the fact that it's fat-soluble (unlike vitamin C, e.g., which is water-soluble). Consequently, vitamin E is exceedingly valuable in protecting cell membranes (which are fatty in composition) from oxidative damage caused by free radicals. By helping to keep the membranes healthy, vitamin E helps keep the entire cell healthy as well. But its benefits go well beyond that.

*Actually, vitamin E is not a single compound, but a group of eight closely related compounds: four tocopherols and four tocotrienols. All eight have biological activity, but the most active one is alpha-tocopherol. Another one, gamma-tocopherol, may contribute significantly to human health in ways that have not yet been recognized.

All the body's tissues contain lipids (fats and other fatty compounds), but the brain is especially rich in these vital substances, which are highly susceptible to oxidative damage from free radicals. The brain therefore requires a great deal of antioxidant protection - all the more so because it consumes a disproportionate amount of the body's oxygen supply, making it that much more vulnerable to oxidative damage. Not surprisingly, recent research suggests that increased intake of vitamin E helps preserve brain function and protect against neuronal (nerve-cell) degeneration. In essence, a healthy intake of vitamin E can prevent or slow the rate of cognitive decline as the brain ages.

A healthy intake of vitamin E can prevent or slow the rate of cognitive decline as the brain ages.

Vitamin E Retards Cognitive Decline

Researchers in Chicago performed a study on 2889 older individuals (aged 65-102, with an average age of 74) to determine whether antioxidants in their diet protect against age-related cognitive decline.2 They determined the typical dietary intake of the participants, calculated their specific intake of antioxidants, and performed a variety of neuropsychological tests to evaluate the participants' cognitive abilities at the beginning and end of the study (the average follow-up period was 3.2 years).

The researchers investigated the potential neuroprotective effects of several antioxidants, including vitamin E, vitamin C, and beta-carotene (a precursor of vitamin A). Only one of these nutrients, however - vitamin E - was found to protect significantly against cognitive decline. There was only a weak link between the rate of cognitive decline and vitamin C intake, and no link at all with beta-carotene intake. (Although beta-carotene and other vitamin A precursors have antioxidant activity in laboratory experiments, they do not generally show this activity in actual human bodies.)


High antioxidant intake may delay the onset of dementia. Vitamin E's ability to protect neurons may thus have an important bearing on healthy neurological aging.

Your Mind Could Be 8-9 Years Younger

The Chicago researchers analyzed their data in two different ways - first by looking at the amount of vitamin E from food sources only, and second by considering the total vitamin E intake from both food and supplements. With both approaches, the conclusion was the same:

those individuals with the highest intake of vitamin E exhibited the least cognitive decline. Specifically, when subjects in the highest quintile (the highest one-fifth, 20%) of vitamin E intake were compared to those in the lowest quintile, the former group was found to have had a 36% reduction in the rate of cognitive decline compared with the latter group.

The researchers reached this startling conclusion:

Vitamin E intake from foods and supplements was associated with reduced cognitive decline in this older biracial population. . . . The effects on cognitive decline in the highest quintiles of vitamin E intake (total or from foods only) were equivalent to a corresponding decrease in age of 8 to 9 years.

In other words, just by maintaining a high intake of vitamin E from food alone, it was possible to avoid the equivalent of an 8-to-9-year cognitive aging effect caused by a low intake of this vitamin. The supplement users' 33-fold higher intake of vitamin E (in the highest quintile of that group) conferred no additional advantage. Does that mean that supplementation with vitamin E has no value? Certainly not! If you are not in the highest quintile of vitamin E intake from food alone (and 80% of the population is, by definition, not in that quintile), supplementation would have definite value. Besides, there is much more to vitamin E than its effect on cognitive function, as we will see below.

Vitamin E May Combat Dementia

Given the important role that vitamin E evidently plays in protecting cognitive function, there is hope that supplementation with this vitamin may help in preventing, or at least delaying the onset of, serious neurodegenerative disorders, such as Alzheimer's and Parkinson's diseases. Alzheimer's research is particularly promising in this area, and several studies suggest that high antioxidant intake may delay the onset of dementia. The ability of vitamin E to protect neurons against oxidative damage may thus have an important bearing on healthy neurological aging.

The value of vitamin E does not stop at the brain, of course. It has long been known that other parts of the body - especially the heart - benefit greatly from higher levels of this vital nutrient.

### Vitamin E Is Good for the Heart

Because vitamin E is fat-soluble, its antioxidant action occurs mainly on lipids, and it appears to play an especially important role in limiting the oxidation of LDL-cholesterol ("bad cholesterol"). When LDL is oxidized, it becomes chemically "stickier," in a sense, and this promotes its accumulation, as plaque, inside our arteries. That, of course, leads to atherosclerosis, a major risk factor for heart disease and stroke. Additional data suggest that vitamin E may also prevent the thickening of blood-vessel walls and at the same time enable them to dilate more easily, thus permitting the freer flow of blood (at a lower blood pressure).3 Improvement in all these conditions favors good cardiovascular health - and in the brain, good cerebrovascular health.

Modest vitamin E supplementation significantly decreases the risk of heart attack. Vitamin E was particularly beneficial for women, decreasing the risk by 34%.

Vitamin E also inhibits platelet aggregation* and may thus serve to inhibit thrombosis (clot formation), which could lead to a heart attack or stroke by limiting blood flow to the heart or brain. Studies conducted in both men4 and women5 have demonstrated that modest vitamin E supplementation (100 IU/day) for more than 2 years significantly decreases the risk of heart attack. Vitamin E was particularly beneficial for women, decreasing the risk of heart attack by 34%. Interestingly, the risk could be decreased even further - to 53% - in combination with vitamin C supplementation, presumably because of vitamin C's ability to regenerate vitamin E in what is known as the "antioxidant network."

*Inhibition of platelet aggregation is generally considered to be good, and agents that have this effect are called anticoagulants, or blood thinners. If two such agents are taken at the same time, however, their effects may be additive. Those who are taking anticoagulant drugs such as heparin or warfarin should consult their doctor before supplementing their diets with large amounts of vitamin E.

### Vitamin E - Good for the Whole Body

Vitamin E was discovered 80 years ago, in 1922. Today, this essential nutrient is widely regarded as a vital antioxidant that protects cell membranes and other lipid structures from oxidative damage. Its benefits are widespread, from the heart to the brain to every other tissue in the body. In your quest to improve your quality of life, be sure to pay particular attention to vitamin E. Make sure the amount you ingest is adequate not only to sustain normal cellular functions but also to help protect those two vital organs - the heart and the brain - that need it most.


Dr. Jensen is a cell biologist who has conducted research in England, Germany, and the United States. He has taught college courses in biology and nutrition and has written extensively on medical and scientific topics.


Vitamin C


Bebrainfit.com reports on vitamin C;


Neurotransmitter Production

Your brain has approximately 100 billion neurons which communicate with each other via brain chemicals called neurotransmitters. Vitamin C is essential in their production. Neurotransmitters impact your ability to focus, concentrate, and remember. They also control your mood, cravings, addictions, sleep, and more. Improved Mood, vitamin C can make you happy! In a recent study, subjects randomly given vitamin C reported feeling happier, often within as little as one week. Vitamin C specifically increases the neurotransmitter serotonin, the "happy molecule," it may act as nature's own natural antidepressant.

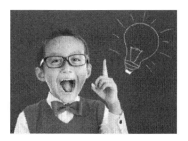

A little boy with a big idea "It's smart to take vitamin C, and it may make you even smarter," states bestselling author Jean Carper in Your Miracle Brain.

Vitamin C supplements can improve IQ, memory and other mental functions.

Students with the highest blood levels of vitamin C did better on memory tests, but higher amounts of vitamin C can boost brain function at all ages.

# Chapter 6
# Supplements

## My Daily Regimen of Supplements

| Omega 3, 6, 9 | 1000 iu | 1 | morning |
|---|---|---|---|
| Coconut Oil | 4   g | 6 | 3 morning 3 evening |
| Turmeric | 800 mg | 2 | 1 morning 1 evening |
| Melatonin | 10 mg | 1 | evening |
| Vinpocetine | 5 mg | 1 | evening |
| Magnesium Complex | 400 mg | 1 | evening |
| Huperzine A | 100 mg | 1 | evening |
| Lion's Mane | 1   g | 3 | evening |

# Omega 3, 6, 9

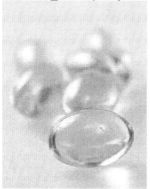

Omega-3 Fatty Acids Increase Brain Volume
While Reversing Many Aspects of Neurologic Aging
August 2010
By Julius Goepp, MD

The cardio-protective power of omega-3 fatty acids has been thoroughly documented in clinical literature. Less well known is their paramount role in optimizing many facets of brain function, from depression, cognition, and memory to mental health.

Recent research has opened up a new horizon in our understanding of omega-3s' profound ability to halt age-related decline and pathology, shattering the long-held medical belief that brain shrinkage and nerve cell death is progressive and irreversible. Omega-3s have been shown to possess antidepressant and neuroprotective properties. One recent landmark study found that aging humans who consumed more omega-3s had increased gray matter brain volume and that most new tissue development was observed in the part of the brain associated with happiness.

Similar findings appeared in the prestigious journal Lancet.2 In one of the largest studies of its kind, scientists analyzing the diets of 12,000 pregnant women found that children of those who consumed the least omega-3 were 48% more likely to score in the lowest quartile on IQ tests.

In this article, the latest research on these essential fatty acids' importance to the growth, development, and function of the human brain is detailed. You will learn about their intrinsic power to preserve cognition and memory and reverse age-related loss of brain function. You will also discover exciting findings on their unique capacity to combat multiple forms of mental illness, neuropsychiatric disorders, and aberrant behavior, from Alzheimer's disease and aggression to bipolar disorder and depression.

Key Nutrient from the Cradle to the Grave

Approximately 8% of the brain's weight is comprised of omega-3 fatty acids3—the building block for an estimated 100 billion neurons. Docosahexaenoic acid (DHA) and eicosapentaenoic acid (EPA) play a host of vital roles in neuronal structure and function, protecting them from oxidative damage, inflammation, and the cumulative destruction inflicted by other chronic insults.

Embedded in the omega-3-rich neuronal membrane are numerous proteins and complex molecules required for electrochemical transmission and signal reception. Scientists have recently shown that the precise balance of fatty acids in brain cells helps determine whether a given nerve cell will be protected against injury or inflammation, or whether it will instead succumb to the injury.7

Omega-3s accumulate in the human brain during fetal development. The amount of the omega-3 DHA has been closely tied to intelligence and cognitive performance in infancy and childhood.8 But the omega-3 content of brain cell membranes involved in essential memory-processing areas diminishes with advancing age and in certain chronic brain disorders.

These findings have led scientists to suspect a role for omega-3 deterioration in development of typical age-related cognitive decline such as that seen in Alzheimer's and chronic disease.

Early developmental deficits in brain content of omega-3s have been associated with poor brain maturation and neurocognitive dysfunction. These are manifested especially in the area of attention, increasing the risk for attention-deficit/hyperactivity disorder (ADHD) and other behavioral disturbances. Later in life, declining levels of DHA and EPA may contribute to development of aggression, anxiety, depression, schizophrenia, dementia, and a variety of other mental health and even criminal conditions.

Scientists are having great success at reversing many of the fundamental age-related decreases in brain function correlated with omega-3 deficiency. ADHD and related conditions can be prevented or mitigated by supplementing infants and nursing mothers with DHA. Young rats supplemented with DHA show increased plasticity or flexibility of function, in their developing brain cells, with highly invigorated development of synapses, the electrochemical junctions where nerve signals are relayed. In aged rats, omega-3 supplementation reverses age-related neuronal changes and maintains learning and memory performance that arise from powerful antioxidant and anti-inflammatory effects.

A remarkable animal study has just revealed that omega-3 fatty acids halt the age-related loss of brain cell receptors vital to memory production, and show potential for increasing neuronal growth.

## Omega 3 is a natural crime fighter!

Recent findings suggest that some criminal and aggressive behaviors are closely correlated with low serum omega-3 levels, which are linked to lower levels of altruism, honesty, and self-discipline. These effects may be related to alterations in serotonin turnover, which controls impulsivity and aggression-hostility behaviors.

There's solid data indicating that optimal omega-3 intake at all ages is a promising avenue for subduing aggression and hostility. For example, 1.5 grams of omega-3 supplementation (containing 840 mg EPA and 700 mg of DHA) in autistic children with severe tantrums, aggression, or self-injurious behavior produced significant improvements compared with placebo, without adverse effects. And stressed but otherwise healthy volunteers given 1,500 mg/day of DHA reported a significantly improved rate of stress reduction compared to a no-treatment group, suggesting an adaptogenic role for omega-3s (adaptogens help the body respond to imposed stress in a variety of ways).

In a group of substance abusers, supplementation with 2,225 mg EPA and 500 mg DHA for 3 months produced significant decreases in anger and anxiety scores compared to placebo recipients. Amazingly, the two nutrients complemented each other, with EPA increases being most robustly associated with lowered anxiety scores, and DHA increases with lowered anger scores. Similarly, in young adult prison inmates, multi-supplements featuring omega-3s produced significant reductions in antisocial, violent, aggressive, and transgressive (rule-breaking) behavior.

More Potent than Prozac®

Large epidemiological studies repeatedly demonstrate that depressed people have significantly reduced levels of DHA and EPA in red blood cell membranes or serum. One autopsy study revealed lower amount of omega-3s in the brains of those who'd suffered depression compared to those who did not. Low omega-3 status is frequently found in people who have attempted or committed suicide. In fact, seasonal variations in blood levels of omega-3s have been shown to closely parallel similar variations in violent suicide deaths. Patients with deficient omega-3 status also had reduced expression of the vital transporter complex responsible for moving serotonin at nerve cell junctions.

People who get more omega-3s actually have bigger, more functional brains.

In fact, the serotonin-related benefits of omega-3 supplementation are powerful enough to stand up to a head-to-head comparison with fluoxetine (Prozac®), a common and highly effective member of the selective serotonin reuptake inhibitor (SSRI) category of modern antidepressants. In that study, 50% of subjects responded well to fluoxetine alone, 56% to EPA supplementation (1,000 mg), and an impressive 81% in people who took both forms of treatment.

## WHAT YOU NEED TO KNOW: REVERSE BRAIN AGING

• Lipids comprise a significant portion of the brain. Of these lipids, omega-3 fatty acids are particularly important.

• Omega-3 fatty acids exert profound anti-aging effects on brain structure and function, from cognition and memory to mental health and Alzheimer's prevention.

• They have recently been associated with increased volume of the brain's gray matter, especially in those regions associated with happiness, and they boost intelligence through enhanced function from birth onwards.

• They support brain cell structure, increase the production of vital neurotransmitters, and blunt oxidative and inflammatory damage.

• Ranges of 1,000-3,000 mg of EPA and 1,000-1,500 mg of DHA have been shown to yield significant improvements in symptoms of depression, aggression, and other mental disorders, as well as protection against early cognitive decline and even early Alzheimer's disease.

At doses above 2,000 mg, results are uniformly dramatic. Double-blind, placebo-controlled trials are revealing substantial superiority of omega-3 therapy to placebo, using standard depression assessment scales. Numerous other studies are further validating these dramatic effects on depression in a host of other contexts: depressive symptoms were alleviated in patients with Parkinson's disease, and in pregnant women with major depressive disorder. A particularly powerful effect was shown in middle-aged women experiencing psychological distress and depressive symptoms during the menopausal transition. In one Israeli study, omega-3 supplementation in children with major depression provided significant improvement across all indices of measurement.

# Coconut Oil

This part of the section I like... Coconut oil, I found clear changes with its use and relatively quickly too. Don't short cut by leaving something out, but be patient when you start taking coconut oil and figure within 60 – 90 days you will begin to notice some positive changes. There were times that I ran out of it and within a few days I was somewhat worse. Once back on the coconut oil, I was feeling better again. I am not sure if better is the right word here, as it suggest all better. I was not, at least, not just from coconut oil. There were clear positive changes. I take 3 soft gels in the morning and 3 every night.

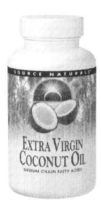

Bebrainfit.com

**An Evidence-Based Look at Coconut Oil and Dementia**
By Deane Alban

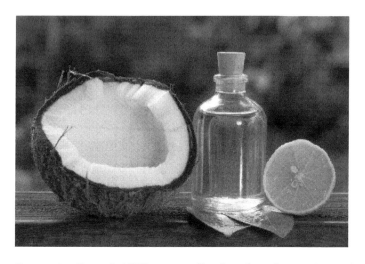

Coconut oil and MCTs are effective for dementia and Alzheimer's. And using coconut oil instead of vegetable oils protects your brain from degenerative disease.

In the past few years coconut oil has experienced a reversal of fortune.

It's gone from being considered an unhealthy fat to being the latest superfood.

In countries of Asia and the South Pacific where coconut is called the "tree of life," it never went out of fashion.

Populations that traditionally use coconut oil are exceptionally healthy with low incidences of modern diseases like heart disease, cancer, and diabetes.

Now the rest of the world is finally coming back around!

One potential use for coconut oil that's still under debate is as a treatment for dementia and Alzheimer's.

There is convincing anecdotal evidence that coconut oil can halt and even reverse the progression of degenerative brain diseases.

But does this hold up to scientific scrutiny?

And if not, should you include coconut oil in your diet anyway?

Here's everything you need to know about how coconut oil uniquely feeds the brain and how effective it is for preventing and treating dementia and Alzheimer's.

How important it is for you in maintaining a healthy brain?

Your Brain Needs Healthy Dietary Fats

First, let's get this out of the way.

Low-fat diets have been a disaster for our brains.

Some experts believe low-fat eating may be responsible for the recent increase in brain disorders such as anxiety, depression, ADHD, and even Alzheimer's.

Of all your organs, your brain especially needs fat.

It's largely made up of fat, 60% by weight.

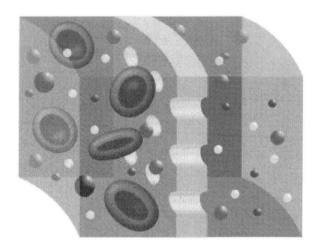

Your brain cell membrane integrity largely depends on the quality of the fats you eat.

And healthy brain cell membranes are critical for brain health and function.

They control what's allowed in (nutrients) and what gets out (toxins).

When unhealthy trans fats get integrated into brain cell membranes, they become less efficient.

Trans fats even condemn your brain cells to shorter lives.

It's not an exaggeration to say the quality of your brain cells depend on the quality of the fats you eat.

The healthiest plant-based fats are not canola, soy, sunflower, and other seed-based oils like we've been led to believe.

They are highly processed and easily turn into unhealthy trans fats once heated or exposed to air but foods that contain fats that are good for your brain; include avocados, nuts, fatty cold-water fish and olive oil. When it comes to healthy brain foods, coconut oil is in a category of its own.

Here's why.

How Medium Chain Triglycerides Uniquely Feed the Brain

There are few dietary sources of medium chain triglycerides (MCTs), and the best source by far is coconut oil.

MCTs are critical for the development of the human brain and are found in abundance in breast milk.

People who cook with coconut oil get plenty of MCTs, but they are rare in the typical modern diet.

Most vegetable oils are long chain triglycerides.

These are larger molecules that are hard to break down and are readily stored as fat.

Coconut oil's unique medium chain triglycerides are smaller; more easily broken down, and are available as a backup source of energy for your brain.

Here's why that's important:

Your brain uses 20% of your daily energy input.

Your brain does not store energy so it needs a constant supply.

For most people, most of the time energy is provided in the form of blood glucose.

If your brain cells don't get the energy they need, they start to die within minutes.

Fortunately, there's a back-up energy system in place for times you can't get the energy your brain needs from carbohydrates.

Your liver breaks down stored fat to produce ketones (also called ketone bodies) that can be used as a substitute fuel during times of starvation.

Ketones readily cross the blood-brain barrier to provide instant energy to brain cells.

Normally there aren't a lot of ketones in the body to provide energy to the brain.

One way to access ketones as an alternative source of brain fuel is with a high-fat, low-carb ketogenic diet.

Ketogenic diets have been used to treat children with epilepsy for decades.

But not everyone wants to eat this way and it is notoriously difficult to get people with dementia or Alzheimer's to change their diets.

Coconut oil and its MCTs provide a convenient workaround.

They provide instant energy to brain cells without the assistance of insulin.

Here's why that's key to understanding how coconut oil can help dementia and Alzheimer's.

Alzheimer's: Diabetes of the Brain

What does this ability of MCTs to fuel the brain without insulin have to do with Alzheimer's?

As we age, our brains become less able to process glucose as brain fuel.

Brain cells can become insulin-resistant.

Alzheimer's patients' brain cells have lost the ability to uptake the glucose they need and subsequently die.

This has led to the theory that Alzheimer's is actually a type of diabetes — diabetes of the brain.

It's sometimes referred to as type 3 diabetes.

But coconut oil bypasses glucose metabolism, getting energy directly to the brain cells that need it.

By using PET scans, it can be seen that the areas of the brain affected by Alzheimer's readily take up ketones as an alternative fuel source.

This is very exciting news!

Dementia and Alzheimer's are often used interchangeably, but are not the same thing. Dementia is an umbrella terms that describes a set of symptoms. There are over 90 types of dementia. Alzheimer's is one of them.

The Alzheimer's Case that Put Coconut Oil on the Map

As a neonatal physician, Dr. Mary Newport was very familiar with the use of MCT oil supplements which are given to premature infants.

When her husband, Steve, developed early-onset Alzheimer's she understood how the MCTs in coconut oil could bypass glucose metabolism to directly feed his brain.

She included coconut oil in his diet along with supplemental MCT oil with considerable success.

One standard measurement for Alzheimer's and other neurological disorders is the Clock-Drawing Test.

Patients are asked to draw a clock.

If their clock is missing important details like hands or numbers, it's indicative of a problem.

Steve took the clock test before starting his coconut oil regime and then again shortly thereafter.

Here are his results.

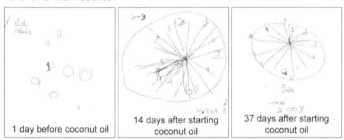

1 day before coconut oil | 14 days after starting coconut oil | 37 days after starting coconut oil

You can see how his clock renderings dramatically improved after a short time on coconut oil indicating his brain function was improving.

Dr. Newport wrote a detailed account of her husband's progress and her struggle to get the medical establishment to consider coconut oil and MCT oil treatment in Alzheimer's Disease: What If There Was a Cure? .

In her book, you'll note that her husband's progress was not all uphill.

Over the years he has experienced ups and downs.

But Dr. Newport is certain that coconut oil slowed down the progression of his disease.

Dr. Newport's Coconut Oil Recommendations for Dementia

Dr. Newport recommends starting with 1 teaspoon of coconut oil 2 or 3 times a day with food and working up to 3 to 5 tablespoons a day of coconut oil and/or MCT oil.

Signs you've taken too much too soon are diarrhea or an upset stomach.

Dr. Newport reports that coconut oil is now being successfully used for treating many neurological disorders including Parkinson's, stroke, traumatic brain injury, glaucoma, Down syndrome, amyotrophic lateral sclerosis, and Huntington's.

It also reduces diabetic complications such as insulin resistance, retinopathy and kidney damage.

Dr. Newport has been contacted by hundreds of people who have halted or even reversed their mental decline with coconut oil.

The growing body of anecdotal evidence for coconut oil for Alzheimer's and other neurological disorders is compelling.

But anecdotal evidence for using coconut oil to treat dementia is not enough for the practice to be endorsed by the mainstream medical community.

# Turmeric

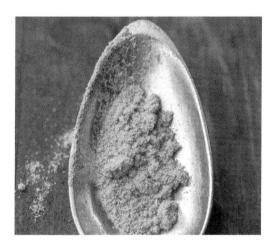

I am sure you have been hearing about Turmeric of late. I have been taking in for some time now and do suggest you read as much as you can about the spice.

The following was taken from greenmedinfo.com.

Long considered impossible to accomplish, new research reveals how a simple spice might contribute to the regeneration of the damaged brain.

Turmeric is hands down one of the, if not the, most versatile healing spice in the world with over 600 experimentally confirmed health benefits, and an ancient history filled with deep reverence for its seemingly compassionate power to alleviate human suffering.

But, most of the focus over the past decade has been centered on only one of its many hundreds of phyto-compounds: namely, the primary polyphenol in turmeric known as curcumin which gives the spice its richly golden hue. This curcumin-centric focus has led to the development of some very good products, such as phospholipid bound curcumin concentrate (e.g. Meriva, BCM-95) which greatly helps to increase the absorption and bio-activity of curcumin. But, curcumin isolates are only capable of conferring a part of turmeric's therapeutic power – and therein lays the limitation and hubris of the dominant 'isolate the active ingredient' model.

Indeed, it has become typical within the so-called nutraceutical industry to emulate the pharmaceutical model, which focuses on identifying a particular "mono-chemical" tree within the forest of complexity represented by each botanical agent, striving to standardize the delivery of each purported 'active ingredient' with each serving, as if it were a pharmaceutical drug. These extraction and isolation processes also generates proprietary formulas which are what manufacturers want to differentiate their product from all others and henceforth capture a larger part of the market share; a value proposition that serves the manufacturer and not the consumer/patient.

Truth be told, there is no singular 'magic bullet' in foods and herbs responsible for reproducing the whole plant's healing power. There are, in fact, in most healing plants or foods hundreds of compounds orchestrated by the intelligent 'invisible hand' of God or 'Nature,' or whatever you wish to call it, and which can never be reduced to the activity of a singularly quantifiable phytocompound or chemical.

# Melatonin

This was suggested to me later in my process and did notice positive results and continue to take it daily. Melatonin is a hormone made by the pineal gland, a small gland in the brain. Melatonin helps control your sleep and wake cycles. Very small amounts of it are found in foods such as meats, grains, fruits, and vegetables. You can also buy it as a supplement.

After about a week of adding the Melatonin, I started meditating. At first I would meditate a few minutes every 3 or 4 days and was trying to find my place with it.

- Extra Strength
- Healthy Sleep Cycle
- Free Radical Scavenger
- Gastrointestinal Support
- Vegetarian/Vegan
- Non-GMO

Melatonin is a potent free radical scavenger naturally produced in the pineal gland and present in high amounts in the gastrointestinal tract. It is involved in many of the body, brain and glandular biological functions including regulation of normal sleep/wake cycles, regulation of the immune system and maintenance of a healthy gastrointestinal lining.

Lifeextention.com reports;

Melatonin: The Brain Hormone
September 2013
By Stephen Fredericks

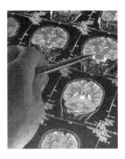

Melatonin was introduced to the United States in 1992 as a "sleep hormone."
While some find melatonin helps restore restful sleep, scientists are finding far more consistent applications for melatonin in the area of brain protection.

New discoveries are validating melatonin's ability to guard the brain from oxidative stress and the neurodegeneration that occurs as a result of aging and environmental factors. With this research, melatonin deserves the title of "brain hormone."

Scientists are increasingly finding that the age-related decline in melatonin levels may be one factor for the age-related increase in neurodegenerative diseases. In fact, some symptoms of melatonin deficiency are seen in patients with Alzheimer's, such as disruption of day/night patterns, mood changes, and delirium.

Fortunately, supplementing with melatonin in middle age and beyond has been shown to protect against Alzheimer's as well as reduce the risk of Parkinson's disease, shrink the size of the infarct area involved in a stroke, and minimize the brain swelling and dysfunction following a head injury.

As if this were not enough, research is also finding that in lab studies melatonin can play a role in longevity by increasing the "longevity protein" SIRT1. Clearly, melatonin's beneficial properties extend far beyond sleep.

## Melatonin's Role in Neurodegenerative Diseases

Some scientists think the increase in neurodegenerative diseases as we age may be directly related to the age-related decline in melatonin levels.[2-4] Fortunately, oral melatonin supplements are available, which may combat this decline by increasing blood and brain levels of melatonin.

Supplementation with low-cost melatonin thus offers an opportunity to restore the brain's natural antioxidant protection and potentially prevent age-related changes to the brain.[2,4,6,16,17] In fact, melatonin's effects are so powerful that it's been designated a drug by the European Medicines Agency (EMA).

With the onset of menopause, animals (like humans) experience a marked increase in oxidative damage, leading to brain cell dysfunction.[18] Studies show that in such animals, melatonin supplementation reverses those harmful effects in a similar manner to hormone replacement—but without the associated risks.

## Melatonin Deficiency Linked to Alzheimer's disease

Melatonin deficiency and Alzheimer's disease are closely linked; profound reductions in melatonin levels have been found in Alzheimer's disease patients. Melatonin, which is maintained at high levels in the brain and spinal fluid throughout youth and middle age, begins to decline sharply with advancing age—in a fashion that closely parallels the rise of Alzheimer's incidence.

One impressive study found that melatonin levels in the spinal fluid of adults older than 80 were just half those of younger, healthy individuals. 21 But older adults who had Alzheimer's had dramatically lower levels yet—roughly one-fifth of those in healthy young people.

This connection is often overlooked, but vitally important—especially because some of the symptoms that arise as a result of melatonin deficiency are detected long before other more obvious cognitive Alzheimer's symptoms present themselves. This makes melatonin deficiency one of the earliest indicators of Alzheimer's disease.

Most notably, these include symptoms such as insomnia and sundowning. Sundowning is a "circadian" (daily rhythm) disturbance in which agitation and activity increase, rather than slow down, as the day wanes. Sleep disorders (such as insomnia, restlessness, and poor sleep quality) generally increase with age and are a sign of declining melatonin production. Such disorders occur in about 45% of those with Alzheimer's.

Fortunately, clinical research has demonstrated the value of melatonin supplementation in reversing these and other changes associated with Alzheimer's, particularly when implemented early in the course of the disease.

## Melatonin Fights Brain Changes in Alzheimer's Disease

In animals given the drug haloperidol (Haldol®), which impairs melatonin synthesis, memory deficits and brain protein changes resembling Alzheimer's disease arise. However, when the animals are then supplemented with melatonin, the changes disappear, indicating a critical role for melatonin in protecting neurons.

In addition, melatonin has been found to help combat Alzheimer's disease by reducing the damage caused by two harmful proteins: amyloid beta proteins and tau proteins. High levels of these two proteins contribute to the death of brain cells and have been linked to Alzheimer's disease.

Melatonin also helps fight Alzheimer's disease by guarding against the harmful effects of aluminum, which is known to produce Alzheimer's-like oxidative changes in brain cells.

Together, these biochemical effects help to explain why melatonin supplementation has been found to reduce learning and memory deficits in animal models of Alzheimer's disease.

## Why It's Important to Start Melatonin Early

Researchers agree that it's best to start taking melatonin before symptoms arise and before physical changes in brain cells have occurred.

One particular animal study demonstrated just how dramatic melatonin's preventive properties really are. For the study, scientists used mice that had human genes predisposed to Alzheimer's disease (these are called transgenic mice).

By late-middle age, the un-supplemented mice proceeded to develop the behavioral and cognitive deficits typical of the disease. In fact, even before signs of disease were visible, the animals' brains already manifested the typical increased oxidation and decreased intracellular antioxidant defenses seen in Alzheimer's. Soon their brain cells began to die off.

However, mice that were supplemented with melatonin before any disease was evident showed none of those pathological changes—and they performed normally on cognitive and behavioral tests.

This shows just how powerfully melatonin works as a preventive agent. Unfortunately, it's been difficult to prove these preventive benefits in people because human trials of interventions for Alzheimer's tend to start only after the disease has become apparent—and well after the window of opportunity for intervention has closed. Nonetheless, very encouraging findings come from studies showing that Alzheimer's patients taking melatonin experience improved sleep patterns, less sun downing, and slower progression of cognitive impairment. Even more evidence that it's best to start melatonin supplements as early as possible comes from several recent studies of mild cognitive impairment, a condition defined as impairment that precedes actual dementia. About 12% of people with mild cognitive impairment proceed to develop dementia each year. In a series of studies, researchers have now shown that people taking between 3 and 24 mg of a fast-acting formulation of melatonin daily for 15 to 60 months performed significantly better on a host of cognitive assessment scales and tests of memory.

## WHAT YOU NEED TO KNOW

Melatonin: The Brain Hormone

•       Melatonin, a hormone produced in the pineal gland of the brain, is well known as a sleep aid; it is registered as a drug for that purpose in Europe.

•       Melatonin also has incredible neuroprotective effects.

•       Studies now reveal that melatonin levels begin to decline at just the time when neurodegenerative diseases begin to rise, and there's good scientific evidence for a strong connection between these phenomena.

•       Supplemental melatonin restores normal, youthful levels of the hormone, and provides powerful antioxidant protection for the brain.

•       Laboratory and early clinical studies show that melatonin supplementation can protect against the age-induced brain changes leading to Alzheimer's and Parkinson's diseases, to increased stroke risk, and to susceptibility to brain trauma.
•       To achieve the most benefit from melatonin, begin supplementation as early as possible.

# Vinpocetine

Vinpocetine was suggested by my mother who had done a good amount of research about it. (By the way I have a birth mother who has Alzheimer's and then my mom. Yeah, I am adopted)

Nutrabio.com reports

Vinpocetine

Main Function: Improves brain metabolism by increasing oxygen flow to the brain. Vinpocetine improve memory and mental energy. May improve overall cognitive function, especially memory, concentration, and mental energy. Improves circulation, oxygenation of the blood, and energy utilization in the brain. Also improves vision.

Pronunciation: vinn-PO-seh-teen

Vinpocetine is derived from an alkaloid found in the periwinkle plant. Is has become popular as a memory enhancer and cognitive aid and is used to treat a variety of neurological disorders, including; cerebrovascular disorders – low cerebral blood flow, headache, hypoxia, cerebral atherosclerosis and stroke; mental impairment – poor memory, aphasia, motor disorders, senility and dementias; sensory disorders – hearing impairment, inner-ear problems, dizziness, low visual acuity and diabetic retinopathy; failing neuronal metabolism. Most of these uses have clinical and laboratory support.

Vinpocetine causes dilation of brain blood vessels and it inhibits blood clotting. These actions improve cerebral blood flow, which might explain many of the neurological benefits.

In addition, vinpocetine is thought to increase the absorption of glucose by nerve cells, thereby providing extra energy for the brain. These physiological processes are just beginning to be explored at the molecular level. The fact vinpocetine improves memory and cognition in ailing individuals has led many perfectly healthy people to conclude that it should help them, too – an idea that makes a lot of sense.

## Vinpocetine Is A Powerful Memory Enhancer

Vinpocetine is an oxygenator and activator of cerebral metabolism and as a result it acts as a powerful memory enhancer.

Vinpocetine has been the focus of numerous studies conducted on healthy volunteers to evaluate short and long term memory improvements. The studies reflect how Vinpocetine can help develop and increase intelligence. Vinpocetine has been shown to be particularly effective in functional symptoms such as confusion, loss of attention, lack of concentration, irritability, vertigo, visual and acoustic alterations, and mood changes. Vinpocetine has also been shown to improve cognitive function, and clearly enhances mental lucidity and memory levels.

*Vinpocetine acts on both the circulatory system and the brains metabolism in the following ways:*

1. Vinpocetine passes through the blood brain barrier and increases glucose consumption by brain cells. Glucose is the source of energy for brain cells.

2. Vinpocetine optimizes the Krebs cycle and therefore helps achieve maximum transformation of glucose into energy.

3. Vinpocetine increase levels of oxygenation of the brain cells, and therefore avoiding hypoxias, which usually result in neuronal death.

4. Vinpocetine helps increase the elasticity of erythrocytes, which eases the microcirculation through the brain capillaries and opens up the supply of oxygen and glucose.

5. Vinpocetine works as a cerebral vasodilator helping to improve cerebral blood flow.

6. Vinpocetine may help inhibit platelet aggregation. This stroke as it stops thromboses or blood clots from forming.

Increase elasticity of the erythrocytes helps to reduce the impact that any such clotting could have.

Vinpocetine is a derivative of natural plant extracts and has been used for many years around the world, with proven degrees of efficiency as a powerful memory enhancer.

Vinpocetine improves cerebral blood flow, decreases cerebral vascular resistance and increases cerebral oxygen and glucose utilization. Vinpocetine inhibits phosphodiesterase activity, prevents aggregation and adenosine intake by erythrocytes. Vinpocetine may also suppress disturbances due to hypoxia or to deficient cerebral metabolism.

Vinpocetine is a synthetic derivative of Vincamine and is thought to have a higher degree of potency than Vincamine while exhibiting minimal side effects.

Classification: Oxygenator and Activator of Cerebral Metabolism

IUPAC Name: Eburnamenine-14-carboxylic acid ethylester

Synonyms: Ethyl-apovincaminate, 3, 16 - apovincamininc acid-ethyl-ester

Product Category: Vasodilator and anti-ischemic

Suggested Dosage: 5 mg per day

Reported Uses:

Vinpocetine is reported to exhibit an activity on neuronal metabolism by favoring the aerobic glycolysis and to promote the redistribution of the blood flow towards ischemic areas. Vinpocetine may also act to increase cerebral circulation and the utilization of oxygen, and is commonly cited as an aid to improving memory.

Vinpocetine has been reported as showing promising results in the treatment of tinnitus or ringing of the ears as well as other causes of impaired hearing. Vinpocetine has also been indicated in the treatment of strokes, menopausal symptoms and macular degeneration.

Vinpocetine may act to improve conditions related to insufficient blood flow to the brain including vertigo and Menieres syndrome, difficulty in sleeping, mood changes and depression.

Life-enhancement.com reports as follows;

### Vinpocetine Is Good for Brain Cells

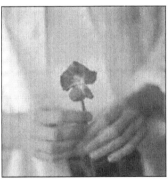

Plant extract may also help restore nerve function in multiple sclerosis

As flowers go, it's pleasant enough - not particularly showy, but with a simple allure. The plant in question is the common periwinkle (Vinca minor), a humble flower whose five petals spiral outward like the spokes of a child's pinwheel, in pink, purple, and violet hues. Simple, pleasant, understated. But that's on the outside. If you take the time to delve deeper, as chemists have, you will discover a rich array of plant compounds with potency that belies the flower's innocent appearance. One of these compounds in particular - vinpocetine - is enriched in the leaves of the plant and has properties that may be important for your health.

Vinpocetine was first isolated and characterized in Hungary about 25 years ago. Early studies with animals demonstrated that vinpocetine significantly increased cerebral blood flow, probably through vasodilation. Put simply, vinpocetine appeared to increase the diameter of blood vessels to the brain, thus increasing its blood supply - and hence the delivery of oxygen and glucose to the brain's cells. It was an exciting result, and raised the question of whether improved blood flow to the brain could improve cognition in humans. It turns out that vinpocetine does indeed have this effect in humans, as evidenced by the results of numerous clinical studies.

VINPOCETINE IS A COGNITIVE ENHANCER

One of the earlier human studies on vinpocetine, conducted in 1987, involved 42 patients with "chronic vascular senile cerebral dysfunction," which means that the patients were suffering from mild-to-moderate dementia caused by cerebrovascular insufficiency, or diminished blood flow to the brain.1 The patients were treated for one month with 10 mg of vinpocetine three times a day, followed by a two-month period of taking 5 mg three times a day. By a variety of measures, vinpocetine improved the general cognition of the patients over this three-month period. In conjunction with other studies, these data helped to establish that vinpocetine improves memory, learning, and speech and language skills in patients suffering from vascular dementia.

There is a veritable mountain of evidence supporting the role of vinpocetine in honing mental abilities. One European database lists over 500 scientific studies on this compound. Not only does vinpocetine enhance mental acuity, it also improves alertness and preparedness skills in cognitively impaired adults. On top of all that, vinpocetine is capable of improving both long-term and short-term memory skills in a range of patients.

*VINPOCETINE IMPROVES BLOOD FLOW TO THE BRAIN*

With respect to cognitive impairment, one researcher claims that "vinpocetine has the most clinical promise for the management of vascular insufficiencies involving the brain."2 This high praise is likely due to the simple fact that vinpocetine improves blood flow to the brain (see the sidebar). As a result, the brain's neurons are well nourished and can respond quickly and adeptly to cognitive challenges.

**How Vinpocetine Works Its Magic**

Strangely enough, vinpocetine is thought to act through the same biological mechanism as sildenafil, the active ingredient in Viagra®. Yet vinpocetine does not appear to have any effect on erectile dysfunction, and sildenafil has not been marketed for improving brain function. So, what's going on here?

Both vinpocetine and sildenafil are biochemically classified as phosphodiesterase inhibitors (PDEIs). Phosphodiesterases (PDEs) are enzymes that come in a variety of forms; at last count there were at least 11 different kinds.1 These protein molecules typically act on smooth muscle tissues, such as those in arterial walls, and prevent them from relaxing. By inhibiting the action of PDEs, PDEIs (such as vinpocetine) allow these tissues to relax, causing dilation of arteries and increasing blood flow to the organs in question.

What's interesting is that different PDEs are present in different tissues. For example, PDE-5 is most common in the penis. Because sildenafil specifically inhibits the action of PDE-5, it enhances blood flow to the penis, thereby facilitating erections.

Vinpocetine, on the other hand, is a PDE-1 inhibitor. PDE-1 is found in the brain, as well as in specific portions of the heart. In the presence of vinpocetine, the brain's arteries dilate and carry more blood, while the rest of the circulatory system is less affected.

*Reference*

1. Truss MC, Stief CG, Uckert S, et al. Initial clinical experience with the selective phosphodiesterase-I isoenzyme inhibitor vinpocetine in the treatment of urge incontinence and low compliance bladder. World J Urol 2000;18:439-43.

Part of vinpocetine's beneficial activity may also be related to its ability to lower the viscosity of blood, i.e., to act as a "blood thinner." It does this by a number of mechanisms. For example, vinpocetine decreases blood-clot formation by lowering the ability of platelets and red blood cells to aggregate. In addition, it makes red blood cells more flexible, which makes them better able to squeeze through tiny capillaries. As a result, blood containing a little vinpocetine is more likely to continue on its journey through the circulatory system unimpeded, and this may partially explain vinpocetine's value in treating other medical conditions.

*VINPOCETINE MAY PROTECT AGAINST ISCHEMIC DAMAGE*

Not only does vinpocetine improve cognition; it may also play a role in protecting the brain's neurons from ischemic injury. Ischemia is a localized loss of blood flow, usually due to blockage of an artery. This condition is especially dangerous in the brain, as neurons are completely dependent on a continuous and ample supply of the oxygen and glucose delivered to them by the blood. Researchers in Portugal have suggested that vinpocetine has antioxidant properties that protect against neuronal damage caused by ischemic injury.[3] Additional laboratory results also suggest that vinpocetine exhibits protective effects against brain ischemia and a protective effect on the brain as a whole, perhaps through its ability to lower the viscosity of blood.

Researchers in Russia undertook a pilot study (a small study to evaluate the desirability and feasibility of conducting a larger clinical trial) on the role of vinpocetine in ischemic stroke patients.4 The results, published recently in the European Journal of Neurology, demonstrated that patients treated with 10 mg of vinpocetine three times a day for three months after their stroke fared marginally better on a National Institute of Health standardized Stroke Scale than the control group. Although there were no statistically significant differences between the treatment and control groups in this or any other measure of the patients' condition, the authors concluded that a large-scale clinical trial should be conducted to investigate more fully the role of vinpocetine in minimizing neuronal damage due to ischemic stroke.

*VINPOCETINE HELPS MS PATIENTS*

Exciting research with vinpocetine has been conducted on patients with multiple sclerosis. MS is a disease in which neural signals from the brain to the target muscle groups are obstructed because sclerotic plaques form in multiple locations along the nerve fibers and interrupt the signal transmission. As a result, the muscles weaken, and MS patients are often tired. In the later stages of the disease, they are often unable to walk, and they lose other motor skills as well.

MS patients treated with phosphodiesterase inhibitors, or PDEIs exhibit a dramatic decrease in relapse rate.5 In a study published in the journal Multiple Sclerosis, 12 patients were treated with a cocktail of three different PDEIs, including 15 mg/day of vinpocetine, for an average of 499 days (1.4 years). The other two ingredients were the anti-Alzheimer's drug propentofylline and the antiasthma drug theophylline.

"Vinpocetine has the most clinical promise for the management of vascular insufficiencies involving the brain."

Before the treatment, the patients averaged 3.1 relapses per year. During the treatment period, however, the incidence of relapses was much lower: only 0.92 per year. Seven of the 12 patients reported no relapses during the treatment period, three had a decreased incidence of relapses, and two had the same incidence as before. Since there were two other ingredients in the treatment formula, one can't say that vinpocetine alone was responsible for these results, but it likely played an important role in reducing the patients' relapse rates.

*VINPOCETINE PROVIDES OTHER BENEFITS*

The benefits of vinpocetine are not limited to the brain. Although vinpocetine does preferentially improve blood flow to the brain, it also increases blood flow to peripheral regions of the body. Two of the organs that benefit greatly from improved blood flow are the eyes and ears (still pretty close to the brain), and the microcirculation in these organs appears to be especially responsive to vinpocetine treatment.

By now you will probably agree that the lowly periwinkle is far from just another pretty face. The next time you walk by this pleasant flower in the garden, see it for what it is: a stunning biological specimen with the ability to restore cognitive powers and sensory perception.

*References*

1.      Balestreri R, Fontana L, Astengo F. A double-blind placebo controlled evaluation of the safety and efficacy of vinpocetine in the treatment of patients with chronic vascular senile cerebral dysfunction. J Am Geriatr Soc 1987;35:425-30.

2.      Kidd PM. A review of nutrients and botanicals in the integrative management of cognitive dysfunction. Altern Med Rev 1999;4:144-61.

3.     Santos MS, Duarte AI, Moreira PI, Oliveira CR. Synaptosomal response to oxidative stress: effect of vinpocetine. Free Radic Res 2000;32:57-66.

4.     Feigin VL, Doronin BM, Popova TF, Gribatcheva EV, Tchervov DV. Vinpocetine treatment in acute ischaemic stroke: a pilot single-blind randomized clinical trial. Eur J Neurol 2001; 8:81-5.

5.     Suzumura A, Nakamuro T, Tamaru T, Takayanagi T. Drop in relapse rate of MS by combination therapy of three different phosphodiesterase inhibitors. Multiple Sclerosis 2000;5:56-8.

# Magnesium Complex

Magnesium Complex  - I take this daily and it is more of a long term accumulative aid. Below is data taken from the web, wellnessresources.com… Once again, for each item I have listed I suggest you do your own research.

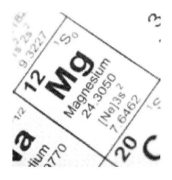

Magnesium Boosts Brain Function
Byron J. Richards, Board Certified Clinical Nutritionist

A study shows that intake of magnesium above what is traditionally considered the normal dietary amount has a dramatic effect on improving multiple aspects of memory and learning. These findings held true for both young and old.

In the study, magnesium directly improved synaptic plasticity, which I previously explained is the key to the future health of your brain. Various regions in the brain associated with learning and memory experienced significant improvements in synaptic function as a result of magnesium dietary supplementation.

A study shows that intake of magnesium above what is traditionally considered the normal dietary amount has a dramatic effect on improving multiple aspects of memory and learning. These findings held true for both young and old.

In the study, magnesium directly improved synaptic plasticity, which I previously explained is the key to the future health of your brain. Various regions in the brain associated with learning and memory experienced significant improvements in synaptic function as a result of magnesium dietary supplementation.

"Our findings suggest that elevating brain magnesium content via increasing magnesium intake might be a useful new strategy to enhance cognitive abilities," explains lead author Guosong Liu, Director of the Center for Learning and Memory at Tsinghua University in Beijing. "Moreover, half the population of industrialized countries has a magnesium deficit, which increases with aging. This may very well contribute to age-dependent memory decline; increasing magnesium intake might prevent or reduce such decline."

The data suggests that the daily recommendation of 400 mg of magnesium, while adequate for some important functions of magnesium, is not adequate for optimal brain function. Over the years I have seen significant health improvement in individuals consuming magnesium in the 600 mg – 1,000 mg range. Because magnesium tends to have a laxative effect the amount any one person can consume as a dietary supplement is sometimes limited by bowel function. However, for those interested in strategies to help maintain optimal brain function, higher levels of magnesium intake are likely to be helpful.

Magnesium is found in fruits and vegetables. However, minerals in food are at low levels due to excessive processing of food, poor farming that depletes soils, and the use of pesticides that interfere with the natural sulfur cycle, leaving us not only with chemically adulterated food but food that has lower nutritional value. It is now common sense to supplement fine quality magnesium.

Quality of magnesium supplements is important. Low quality forms of magnesium include magnesium oxide, magnesium aspartate, magnesium gluconate, and magnesium sulfate. At Wellness Resources, we use highly absorbable, high quality forms of magnesium including magnesium glycinate and magnesium malate.

# Huperzine A

A daily part of my evening dosages is Huperzine A. This was recommended to me a bit later in my process but was not the last... Some if not all of the information that I have taken from the web do have some sales pitch to them... I can only tell you about my experience!

Nootriment.com reports as follows;

Huperzine A Benefits and Effects for Memory and Brain Function

Posted By: Nootriment Editorial Staff

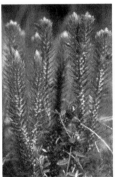

Club moss is a Chinese plant that when purified results in the supplement known as Huperzine A. This natural supplement has a range of nootropic benefits and is known to improve many facets of memory function. The most common uses of Huperzine A include the treatment of neurological problems, such as Alzheimer's disease. It can also be used to aid with the problems that arise from learning deficiencies and memory losses.

Huperzine A benefits and effects arise from the fact that this compound increases acetylcholine levels in the brain. Not only does this increase information retention and memory formation, it can also boost concentration, mental clarity and the ability to process or calculate data.

**How Huperzine A Benefits Your Body**

Huperzine A is an alkaloid and is present naturally in some plants. The most commonly it is extracted from "Chinese Club Moss". Huperzine A is well-known as a food supplement that is of Chinese origin. Most herbalists use huperzine A for the treatment of swelling and fever since old times. Chinese club moss is also one of the herbs which have many active ingredients and these active ingredients are helpful in treating different health related problems.

One of the best known benefits of huperzine A is its effectiveness in treating Alzheimer's disease. Some other benefits of huperzine include memory enhancement, treating muscle fatigue and osteoarthritis.

Some researchers also prescribe huperzine A for increasing memory and learning skills. Individuals, who have been using huperzine A, say that it is very effective in providing relief from muscular fatigue after heavy exercise. Regular use of huperzine A may also increase the amount of acetylcholine in the body. Acetylcholine is a chemical which nerves use for communicating with the muscles, organs and the brain and is very effective for boosting the immune system and it also helps in the communication of the nerves.
Better nervous communication results in increased alertness and memory skills of an individual. Huperzine A may also increase the muscle mass of the individual who regularly uses it as a food supplement. Other than this the plant leaves can also be used as a tea and kehva, Huperzine A may also provide nourishment to the brain cells. Researchers also say that the use of huperzine may also help in preventing the individual from cognitive diseases.

A research carried out by few medical specialists showed that individual who have low levels of huperzine in their body suffered from memory loss. To improve the memory skills huperzine A can be very useful. People who are suffering from dementia may also find huperzine A as a good remedy. People who complain of memory loss and poor thinking skills may find huperzine A very effective. Huperzine A is also effective in preventing the nerves from getting damaged from free radical activities. Huperzine A helps in providing relief during stress and tension both are enemies of Alzheimer's disease and dementia.

# Lion's Mane

**Lion's Mane: A Mushroom That Improves Your Memory and Mood?**

*08/08/2012 08:28 am ET | Updated Oct 08, 2012*

Paul Stamets Founder, Fungi Perfecti; Advisor, Program of Integrative Medicine at the University of Arizona Medical School, Tucson

Mushrooms provide a vast array of potential medicinal compounds. Many mushrooms — such as portobello, oyster, reishi and maitake — are well-known for these properties, but the lion's mane mushroom, in particular, has drawn the attention of researchers for its notable nerve-regenerative properties.

Lion's mane mushrooms are not your classic looking cap-and-stem variety. These globular-shaped mushrooms sport cascading teeth-like spines rather than the more common gills. From these spines, white spores emerge. Lion's mane mushrooms also have other common names: sheep's head, bear's head and the Japanese yamabushitake. I like the clever name "pom pom blanc" — a reference to their resemblance to the white pom-poms cheerleaders use. The Latin name for lion's mane is Hericium erinaceus; both names mean "hedgehog."*

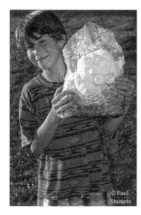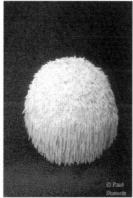

Lion's mane mushrooms are increasingly sold by gourmet food chains. This nutritious mushroom is roughly 20 percent protein, and one of the few that can taste like lobster or shrimp (Stamets, 2005). Lion's mane is best when caramelized in olive oil, deglazed with saké wine, and then finished with butter to taste. Lion's mane can be bitter if not cooked until crispy along the edges. It takes some practice to elicit their full flavor potential.

Lion's mane mushrooms are increasingly studied for their neuroprotective effects. Two novel classes of Nerve Growth Factors (NGFs) — molecules stimulating the differentiation and re-myelination of neurons — have been discovered in this mushroom so far. These cyathane derivatives are termed "hericenones" and "erinacines." The levels of these compounds can vary substantially between strains, based on the measurements our team has conducted.

About a dozen studies have been published on the neuroregenerative properties of lion's mane mushrooms since 1991, when Dr. Kawagishi first identified NGFs in Japanese samples. Since his original discovery, in vitro and in vivo tests have confirmed that hericenones and erinacines stimulate nerve regeneration. In 2009, researchers at the Hokuto Corporation and the Isogo Central and Neurosurgical Hospital published a small clinical study. Giving lion's mane to 30 Japanese patients with mild cognitive impairment resulted in significant benefits for as long as they consumed the mushrooms:

"The subjects of the Yamabushitake group took four 250 mg tablets containing 96 percent of Yamabushitake dry powder three times a day for 16 weeks. After termination of the intake, the subjects were observed for the next four weeks. At weeks eight, 12 and 16 of the trial, the Yamabushitake group showed significantly increased scores on the cognitive function scale compared with the placebo group. The Yamabushitake group's scores increased with the duration of intake, but at week four after the termination of the 16 weeks intake, the scores decreased significantly." (Mori, 2009)

Recently, mice were injected with neurotoxic peptides in an experiment to assess the effects of lion's mane on the type of amyloid plaque formation seen in Alzheimer's patients. The mice were then challenged in a standard "Y" maze, designed for testing memory. Mice fed with a normal diet were compared to those supplemented with lion's mane mushrooms. As the peptide-induced plaque developed, the mice lost the ability to memorize the maze. When these memory-impaired mice were fed a diet containing 5 percent dried lion's mane mushrooms for 23 days, the mice performed significantly better in the Y maze test. Interestingly, the mice regained another cognitive capacity, something comparable to curiosity, as measured by greater time spent exploring novel objects compared to familiar ones.

The reduction of beta amyloid plaques in the brains of mushroom-fed mice vs. the mice not fed any mushrooms was remarkable. The formation of amyloid plaques is what many researchers believe is a primary morphological biomarker associated with Alzheimer's. Plaques linked to beta amyloid peptide inflame brain tissue, interfere with healthy neuron transmission, and are indicated in nerve degeneration.

The medical community is bracing for an increase of patients with Alzheimer's and senile dementia as the baby boomer population ages. Mortality trends related to Alzheimer's are outpacing death rates of many other diseases. This makes preventive and curative treatments of age-related cognitive diseases hot subjects of research. In the past 10 years, deaths from Alzheimer's disease have surged roughly 66 percent, while deaths from other primary diseases have generally declined.

The influence of lion's mane influence on neurological functions may also have other added benefits — making you feel good. In another small clinical study (n=30), post-menopausal women who consumed lion's mane baked into cookies vs. those without showed less anxiety and depression yet improved in their ability to concentrate (Nagano et al., 2010).

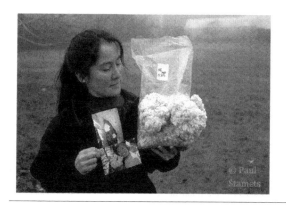

Dusty Yao with lion's mane cultivated three months from the time the wild specimen, featured in photograph, was collected.

Is this data conclusive thus far? No.

Is this data suggestive of positive outcomes? Absolutely.

In another small Japanese study with a randomized sample of 30 women, ingesting lion's mane showed that "HE intake has the possibility to reduce depression and anxiety, and these results suggest a different mechanism from NGF-enhancing action of H. erinaceus." (Nagano et al. 2010).

In light of the numerous diseases related to neurodegeneration, lion's mane deserves more clinical attention. If lion's mane enhances memory and is an antidepressant, can consuming this mushroom alter the course of Alzheimer's and other neurodegenerative diseases? Could this mushroom help Parkinson's patients or those with multiple sclerosis, or maybe maintain your mental acumen as you age? Lion's mane is a relatively inexpensive, easily-cultivated fungal food that may prove to be therapeutic in ways beyond being tasty.

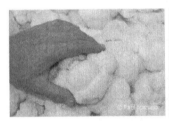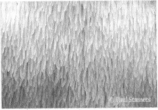

Lion's mane may be our first "smart" mushroom. It is a safe, edible fungus that appears to confer cognitive benefits on our aging population. Unfortunately, lion's mane is not available in most grocery stores. But you can buy kits to grow them at home, and organic lion's mane supplements are available at some health food stores. If you are skilled enough and looking for adventure, you can forage for them by hunting in the hardwood forests of North America, Europe and Asia during the summer and fall.**

Left: Fresh, organically grown lion's mane ready for sale. Right: Close up of spore-producing spines.

*Hedgehog is a name more commonly associated with Hydnum species, specifically the edible Hyndum repandum.

**Before consuming any wild mushroom, make positively sure that it is accurately identified. For a list of mycological societies, which may be able to help you, go to the North American Mycological Association website: www.namyco.org.

References:

Kawagishi, H., Ando, M., Sakamoto, H., Yoshida S., Ojima, F., Ishiguro, Y., Ukai, N., Fukukawa, S. 1991. "Hericenone C, D and E, stimulators of nerve growth factor (NGF) synthesis from the mushroom Hericium erinaceum." Tetrahedron Lett 32, 4561-4564.

Ma, Bing-Ji , Jin-Wen Shen, Hai-You Yu, Yuan Ruan, Ting-Ting Wu & Xu Zhao, 2010. "Hericenones and erinacines: stimulators of nerve growth factor (NGF) biosynthesis in Hericium erinaceus." Mycology: An International Journal on Fungal Biology. 1(2): 92-98.

Mori, K., Inatomi, S., Ouchi, K. Azumi, Y and Tuchida T. 2009. "Improving effects of the mushroom Yamabushitake (Hericium erinaceus) on mild cognitive impairment: a double blinded, placebo controlled clinical trial." Phytother Res. 23:367-372.

Mori, K., Obara, Y., Moriya, T., Inatomi, S., Nakahata, N. 2011. "Effects of Hericium erinaceus on amyloid β(25-35) peptide-induced learning and memory deficits in mice." Biomed Res. 32(1):67-72.

Nagano, M., Shimizu, K., Kondo, R., Hayashi, C., Sato, D., Kitagawa, K., Ohnuki, K. 2010. "Reduction of depression and anxiety by 4 weeks Hericium erinaceus intake." Biomed Res. 31(4):231-7.

Stamets, P., "Notes on nutritional properties of culinary-medicinal mushrooms." International Journal of Medicinal Mushrooms. 2005; 7:109-116.

Thal, L.J., Kantarci, K., Reiman, E.M., Klunk, W.E., Weiner, M.W., Zetterberg, H., Galasko, D., Praticò, D., Griffin, S., Schenk, D., Siemers, E. 2006. "The role of biomarkers in clinical trials for Alzheimer disease." 20(1):6-15.

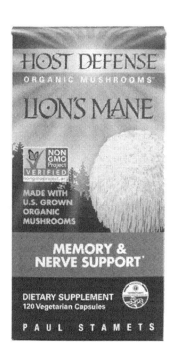

HOST DEFENSE

ORGANIC MUSHROOMS

LION'S MANE

NON GMO Project VERIFIED
nongmoproject.org

MADE WITH U.S. GROWN ORGANIC MUSHROOMS

MEMORY & NERVE SUPPORT*

DIETARY SUPPLEMENT
120 Vegetarian Capsules

PAUL STAMETS

# Chapter 7
# Mental Exercise

## Mental Exercise

I started off naturally doing mental exercise without even realizing it! Trust when I say that I had no idea that I was exercising my brain, but I had always been busy in life. Now I was captive to my illness, and I had to do something with my time. I developed several Facebook friends and socialized online. I would enter comments and start lively debates, nothing nasty, just sharing opinions. I made even more friends as time went by. One who continues learning new things throughout life and challenging his or her brain is less likely to develop Alzheimer's disease and dementia, so make it a point to be mentally active. As in the old saying, you need to "use it or lose it."

As mentioned much earlier within this book I also started writing prior to being diagnosed with Alzheimer's. I never wrote before! It was sort of like my mind was being tickled, and I had to write. I am not sure if that fully conveys what was going on, but at times I was not sure who was holding the pen, so to say!

Then my grandchildren, 7 in all, ranged from young adult on down in age to just about 3 years old. Between conversations with the oldest ones and playing with the younger grandchildren, I was being active. The youngest of whom I had great fun with, oh my did we go on! I did mention him earlier on in the book. In addition to that, when my oldest daughter and I would take a ride together. it was always a hoot. She and I always bantered a lot anyway but even more then! I started playing pranks on everyone as this too is a mental exercise of sorts. You can trust it was all in good fun.

All of the above mentioned are not available to everyone. There are things available at memoryprotocol.com, a memory protocol guide, memory protocol games, and exercises that you might find helpful. I would also suggest crossword puzzles, scrabble, and alike, they are all good mental exercises.

As you can see I had a stress free environment provided by my oldest daughter, lots of love from family and friends. In spite of how I was originally digressing, I had all the support in the world excluding a few bumps in the road, which my daughter fended off. There was a point that I could not draw a clock, it was hard to have a normal conversation with people, I would not speak with anyone outside of family in public, wore a cap 24/7, and slept 15 hours a day. I was a mess! I could not handle anything that took logic and math. I was no longer able to do even simple math. I would lose my place in a verbal conversation and forget where I was going "light not extreme lost". Trust, I am leaving out some of, how bad that bad was. But that was then, and this is now.

Stress can take a heavy toll on the brain, leading to shrinkage in a key memory area of the brain known as the hippocampus, hampering nerve cell growth, and increasing your risk of Alzheimer's disease and dementia. Yet there are simple tools that you can apply to daily life that can minimize the harmful effects of stress.

• Meditate - Most scientists today acknowledge a strong mind-body connection, and various studies associate spirituality with better brain health. Regular meditation, prayer, reflection, and religious practice may immunize you against the damaging effects of stress.
• Learn breathing techniques to quiet the mind.
• Alter how you respond to various situations
• Remove yourself from being around stressful people

- Make time for leisure activities that bring you joy, whether it be stargazing, playing the piano, or working on your bike.
- Play, laugh, and listen to music

## How to Mediate

I use mediation tapes that I have gotten online for free although they can be purchased in spiritual stores, like Earth Spirits in Red Bank NJ. It is best to listen in a dark quiet room. The best way to listen is with headphones on and in a comfortable position. Many people that mediate will sit in a yoga position I personally prefer to lay down. I take about 5 slow deep breaths. There is a yoga breathing technique that is good to learn. With each release of air I relax more from head to toe.

I started off doing this for a few minutes each evening before sleep. Now I do it for hours up to two hours. I end up with a pleasant night's sleep and feel completely refreshed the next day. It's funny I used to mediate some 45 years back and stopped, which was foolish on my part.

## How to Breathe

An easy breathing exercise is to sit comfortably in a chair or on the floor, eyes softly closed, tongue resting gently against the back of the top teeth. Inhale through the nose while counting silently to five. Pause for just a moment, and then exhale for a count of five. Try to keep the breath as even throughout the exercise. Imagine you're sipping air through a straw, which will keep the breath even and flowing. Repeat this exercise several times, until you feel like even inhalations and exhalations are less of an effort. Experiment with longer counts and shorter counts, and notice the effect that each has on your mind and body. What length feels "right" to you?

## Altering your responses

I want to start out by posing two simple questions; do you count your blessings and what are you grateful for? I feel these set the right tone for starting each day.

We have choices to make in any given situation. Most of the time, we listen to react vs listen to learn, so my first suggestion is listen to learn. Listening to learn will cut down the daily volume of stress you face. When we do find we want to respond with an argument, it is best to take your foot and very slightly step back it gives you a moment to think if what you are about to say is worth it. Far too often we speak from a point within our emotions. I will also suggest, and I do this myself, smile! We don't seem to smile enough. Not smiling, or looking unhappy, sets the stage for how people are going to act towards you!

## Remove Stressful people

This is not always easy, but stress is the enemy. I can't say that enough times or firmly enough. Stress really is the bad guy! If someone is creating stress around you; get away from them at all costs. Remember, they are releasing their emotions it has nothing to do with you, but leave their area. If they continue to bring stress into your life literally leave and don't look back. They are not your friend! For you to survive you need peace of mind, relaxation, a harmonic atmosphere around you, and a ton of positive influences in your life. You do not need someone that is always seeing the worst side of life.

## Leisure Activities

What should you do for leisure activities? At our age if you don't know, then you have worked too hard and not played enough! But a simple list may include fishing, bowling, swimming, golf, walks, antiquing, museums, hunt for treasure. These are things that are on my list of things I want to do. Bike riding is another great way to see local sites, plus it is light exercise that is good for you. There is also chess, checkers, scrabble, cards, word games, and reading or better yet writing your memoirs. You might even turn them into a book!

## Music

Music is stored in many areas of the brain and is a basic part of what makes us human, using music associated with personal memories helps reach and engage anyone with dementia and Alzheimer's, even as memory fails. Using personalized music from their life and times can help to connect with love ones at any stage of the disease, improve communication, and increase overall quality of life.

My entire life I have had a love for music. I picked up the guitar at a young age. Sometime after my diagnoses I picked up one of my second oldest grandsons' guitars and started playing, did it ever bring back memories for me. I listen to mediation tapes which are musical, and music is always playing at the gym. They say music soothes the soul, and they also say it music soothes the beast too.

Play music, dance, and laugh! Let the child out to play that you have hidden inside for all these years. Trust me, the kid can't wait!

As I mentioned stress free is important. Caregivers often feel a need to correct the patient, but I am not sure why. The person they are correcting is not the person they used to be, not by a long shot. Actually, in part you are communicating with an adult child and a child that is hurt, confused, and frustrated within their situation! From the perspective that life is over as they knew it, why not make the rest of that life a happy one?

I have to say worry never fixed a thing, and worry leads to unnecessary stress. Stress is the enemy! I can't say that clear enough!

# Chapter 8
# Physical Exercise

Physical Exercise

Before you start exercising speak with you doctor and see what he or she suggests. That being said, for someone with Alzheimer's or dementia exercise is essential. I think I mentioned it before, "trust those enzymes," your spirits will lift gradually over time.

You might start out with simple walks around the block. Set modest goals, and increase them as your body allows. Your exercise program should include the following:

Stretching, which increases blood flow and gets your body ready for exercise. Stretching also improves flexibility, eases movement, and lowers the risk of injury and muscle strain. A warm-up and cool-down period of 5 to 15 minutes should be done slowly and carefully before and after all types of exercise. Stretching can help loosen muscles in the arms, shoulders, back, chest, stomach, buttocks, thighs, and calves. It's also very relaxing. A healthy exercise program should include the following:

Aerobic exercise: Improves cardiovascular fitness and muscle tone. This type of exercise includes activities such as walking, running, swimming, cycling, dancing, rowing, and cross country skiing.

Weight training (resistance) exercise: Promotes muscle strength and flexibility.

Both aerobic and weight training exercise can improve balance. Recent studies have suggested that Tai Chi, an ancient Chinese exercise regimen, may be even more effective than traditional exercise programs in preventing accidental falls in older individuals.

About 2 possibly 3 years ago my oldest daughter and I joined the gym and later my middle daughter also joined.

At first I would walk on the treadmill for maybe 15 minutes. I did not walk fast there was no reason to overdo it. Little by little I increased the time and slightly increased the speed of the walk until I was walking for 30 minutes and left my daughters behind! I had to throw that in...

I not only increased the walk on the treadmill but increased the incline of the walk until I was at the highest level available on the machine. I never did run on it. From that machine I started reaching out to the other exercise equipment that was available, legs, arms, and torso machines.

The torso machine is one that I enjoy using.  I then started using the elliptical machine. On the elliptical I started out the same as the treadmill, 15 minutes and gradually increased the incline.

Today I am in the gym near 2 hours daily and use most the machines available, but never do I overdo it or lift too much. I work out at my own pace. I am there for my enjoyment and enjoy what I do!

Over time at the gym I started making friends. I wore a t-shirt that mentioned that I have Alzheimer's. "If I seem confused and bewildered at times I have Alzheimer's please be kind and smile." Sorry for the blurry image below but it is all I have. They were a support for me at first, but later became a bit of a cheering section, and now friends.

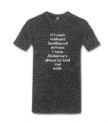

# Chapter 9
# Types of Dementia

**There are 10 different types of Dementia below are some of them.**

There are many conditions which can cause dementia, which makes it vital for the patient to obtain accurate diagnosing of dementia early on so they can receive proper treatment. Following are some of the most common causes and types of dementia.

**Vascular Dementia**
One of the most common forms of dementia, vascular dementia is caused by poor blood flow to the brain, depriving brain cells of the nutrients and oxygen needed to function normally. One of the ten dementia types, vascular dementia can result from any number of conditions which narrow the blood vessels, including stroke, diabetes and hypertension.

**Mixed Dementia**
Sometimes dementia is caused by more than one medical condition. This is called mixed dementia. The most common form of mixed dementia is caused by both Alzheimer's and vascular disease.

**Dementia with Lewy Bodies (DLB)**
Referred to as Lewy Body Disease, this type of dementia is characterized by abnormal protein deposits called Lewy bodies which appear in nerve cells in the brain stem. These deposits disrupt the brain's normal functioning, impairing cognition and behavior and can also cause tremors. DLB is not reversible and has no known cure. It is said that Robin Williams had Lewy Body Dementia.

**Parkinson's disease Dementia (PDD)**

Parkinson's disease is a chronic, progressive neurological condition, and in its advanced stages, the disease can affect cognitive functioning. Not all people with Parkinson's disease will develop dementia, however. Dementia due to Parkinson's is also a Lewy body dementia. Symptoms include tremors, muscle stiffness and speech problems. Reasoning, memory, speech, and judgment are usually affected.

### Frontotemporal Dementia

Pick's disease, is a rare disorder which causes damage to brain cells in the frontal and temporal lobes. Pick's disease affects the individual's personality significantly, usually resulting in a decline in social skills, and emotional apathy. Unlike other types of dementia, Pick's disease typically results in behavior and personality changes manifesting before memory loss and speech problems.

### Creutzfeldt-Jacob Dementia (CJD)

CJD is a degenerative neurological disorder, known as mad cow disease. The incidence is very low, occurring in about one in one million people. There is no cure. Caused by viruses that interfere with the brain's normal functioning, dementia due to CJD progresses rapidly, usually over a period of several months. Symptoms include memory loss, speech impairment, confusion, muscle stiffness and twitching, and general lack of coordination, making the individual susceptible to falls. Occasionally, blurred vision and hallucinations are also associated with the condition.

### Normal Pressure Hydrocephalus (NPH)

Normal pressure hydrocephalus involves an accumulation of cerebrospinal fluid in the brain's cavities. Impaired drainage of this fluid leads to the build-up and results in added pressure on the brain, interfering with the brain's ability to function normally. Individuals with dementia caused by normal pressure hydrocephalus often experience problems with ambulation, balance and bladder control, in addition to cognitive impairments involving speech, problem-solving abilities and memory.

## Huntington's disease

Huntington's disease is an inherited progressive dementia that affects the individual's cognition, behavior and movement. The cognitive and behavioral symptoms of dementia due to Huntington's include memory problems, impaired judgment, mood swings, depression and speech problems (especially slurred speech). Delusions and hallucinations may occur. In addition, the individual may experience difficulty ambulating, and uncontrollable jerking movements of the face and body.

## Wernicke-Korsakoff Syndrome

Wernicke-Korsakoff syndrome is caused by a deficiency in thiamine (Vitamin B1) and often occurs in alcoholics, although it can also result from malnutrition, cancer which have spread in the body, abnormally high thyroid hormone levels, long-term dialysis and long-term diuretic therapy (used to treat congestive heart failure). The symptoms of dementia caused by Wernicke-Korsakoff syndrome include confusion, permanent gaps in memory, and impaired short-term memory. Hallucinations may also occur.

## Mild Cognitive Impairment (MCI)

Dementia may be due to medical illness, medications and a host of other treatable causes. With mild cognitive impairment, individuals will experience loss of memory, often accompanied with impaired judgment and speech, but the person is usually aware of the decline. These problems usually don't interfere with some of the normal activities of daily living. Individuals with mild cognitive impairment may also experience behavioral changes that involve depression, anxiety, aggression and emotional apathy; these can be due to the awareness of and frustration related to his or her condition.

Some of the tests that are commonly used in determining various types of dementia, often given during follow visits to measure progression are;

### Mini Mental State Evaluation (MMSE)
The mini-mental status exam is a very brief evaluation of the patient's cognitive status used in diagnosing dementia types. The patient is required to identify the time, date and place (including street, city and state) where the test is taking place, be able to count backwards, identify objects previously known to him or her, be able to repeat common phrases, perform basic skills involving math, language use and comprehension, and demonstrate basic motor skills.

*Some of the tests that are commonly used in determining various types of dementia, often given during follow visits to measure progression are;*

### Mini Mental State Evaluation (MMSE)

The mini-mental status exam is a very brief evaluation of the patient's cognitive status used in diagnosing dementia types. The patient is required to identify the time, date and place (including street, city and state) where the test is taking place, be able to count backwards, identify objects previously known to him or her, be able to repeat common phrases, perform basic skills involving math, language use and comprehension, and demonstrate basic motor skills.

## Mini-Cog
Another test for diagnosing dementia, the mini-cog takes only a few minutes to administer and it's used as an initial screening for various types of dementia. The patient is required to identify three objects in the office, then draw the face of a clock in its entirety from memory, and finally, recall the three items identified earlier.

## Imaging Tests: CTs, MRIs
Physicians that are diagnosing dementia can study the structure of the patient's brain by CT or MRI to see if there are any growths, abnormalities or general shrinkage (as noted in cases of Alzheimer's).

## As previously mentioned the PET scan
The PET scan provides amazing detail for diagnosing ability

# Chapter 10
# Closing Thoughts

**NEWS ANNOUNCEMENT**

*Amazing news; while this book was in editing the following just came in on a search!*

Anti-Dementia Compounds from Lion's Mane Mushroom the focus of research on medicinal mushrooms until now has been primarily on their anti-cancer and immune-enhancing properties. However, attention has shifted by researchers in Japan and China to the potential anti-dementia properties contained in a mushroom called Lion's Mane (Hericium erinacewn).

A study was done in a rehabilitative hospital in the Gunma prefecture in Japan, with 50 patients in an experimental group and 50 patients used as a control group. All patients suffered from cerebrovascular diseases causing senility, Parkinson's disease, or other spinocerebellar and orthopedic diseases that afflict the elderly. Seven of the patients in the experimental group suffered from different types of dementia. The patients in this group received 5g of dried Lion's Mane Mushroom per day in their soup for a 6-month period. All patients were evaluated before and after the treatment period for Functional Independence Measure (FIM), which is a measure of independence in physical capabilities; eating, dressing, walking, etc., plus their perceptual capacities; understanding, communication, memory, etc.

The results of this preliminary study show that after six months of taking Lion's Mane Mushroom, six out of seven Alzheimer's patients demonstrated improvements in their perceptual capacities, and all seven had improvements in their overall FIM score.

**Just a note**

I have been here after writing all this down and still can't believe what has happened, coming from such a point of darkness. I knew I was improving and that there was no question of that. But my beliefs were confirmed when the seeing the neurologists' mouth drop and I watched his eyes light while saying to me "You have improved" with a happily surprised voice. I have been walking on a cloud since. It could easily be said that I am "stuck in a moment" but this moment of stuck is unbelievably wonderful! I have to be measured about what I say about all of this. I have Alzheimer's disease and I have improved greatly. I can't say I am all better or cured and will not because I am not. What I can say is that I am, dramatically improved and ready to get on with my life.

I am now off of most of the medications excluding donepezil 10 MG twice a day, but I know that too will soon  be downgraded until I am off it all together!

I have been thinking for months about writing this story and where to begin with such an important message to share. I have done my best I hope it helps you!

# Chapter 11
# The Seven Stages

*Alzheimer's symptoms vary from person to person. The seven stages below provide a general idea of how abilities change during the course of the disease.*

Stage 1: No impairment
Stage 2: Very mild decline
Stage 3: Mild decline
Stage 4: Moderate decline
Stage 5: Moderately severe decline
Stage 6: Severe decline
Stage 7: Very severe decline

Not everyone will experience the same symptoms or progress at the same rate. This seven-stage framework is based on a system developed by Barry Reisberg M.D., clinical director of the New York University School of Medicine's Silberstein Aging and Dementia Research Center.

**Stage 1: No impairment** (normal function)

• The person does not experience any memory problems. An interview with a medical professional does not show any evidence of symptoms of dementia.

**Stage 2: Very mild cognitive decline**
(May be normal age-related changes or earliest signs of Alzheimer's)

• The person may feel as if he or she is having memory lapses – forgetting familiar words or the location of everyday objects. But no symptoms of dementia can be detected during a medical examination or by friends, family or co-workers.

**Stage 3: Mild cognitive decline**
(Early-stage Alzheimer's can be diagnosed in some, but not all, individuals with these symptoms)

- Friends, family or co-workers begin to notice difficulties. During a detailed medical interview, doctors may be able to detect problems in memory or concentration.

*Common stage 3 difficulties include:*

- Noticeable problems in coming up with the right word or name.

- Trouble remembering names when introduced to new people.

- Having noticeably greater difficulty in performing tasks in social or work settings.

- Forgetting material that one has just read.

- Losing or misplacing a valuable object.

- Increasing trouble with planning or organizing things.

### Stage 4: Moderate cognitive decline
(Mild or early-stage Alzheimer's)

*At this point a careful medical interview should be able to detect clear symptoms in several areas:*

- Forgetfulness of recent events.

- Impaired ability to perform challenging mental arithmetic – for example, counting backward from 100 by 7s.

- Greater difficulty performing complex tasks, such as planning a dinner for guests, paying bills or managing finances.

- Forgetfulness about one's own personal history.

- Becoming moody or withdrawn, especially in socially or mentally challenging situations.

## Stage 5: Moderately severe cognitive decline
(Moderate or mid-stage Alzheimer's)

- Gaps in memory and thinking are noticeable, and individuals begin to need help with day-to-day activities.

*At this stage, those with Alzheimer's may:*

- Be unable to recall their own address or telephone number, or the high school or college from which they graduated.

- Become confused about where they are or what day it is.

- Have trouble with less challenging mental arithmetic, such as counting backwards from 40 by subtracting 4s or from 20 by 2s.

- Need help choosing proper clothing for the season or occasion.

- Still remember significant details about themselves and their family.

- Require no assistance with eating or using the toilet.

## Stage 6: Severe cognitive decline
(Moderately severe or mid-stage Alzheimer's)

- Memory continues to worsen, personality changes may take place and individuals need extensive help with daily activities.

*At this stage, individuals may:*

- Lose awareness of recent experiences, as well as of their surroundings.

- Remember their own name, but have difficulty with their personal history.

- Distinguish familiar and unfamiliar faces, but have trouble remembering the name of a spouse or caregiver.

- Need help dressing properly and may, without supervision, make mistakes such as putting their pajamas over daytime clothes or putting shoes on the wrong feet.

- Experience major changes in sleep patterns – sleeping during the day and becoming restless at night.

- Need help handling the details of toileting (for example, flushing the toilet, wiping or disposing of tissue properly).

- Have increasingly frequent trouble controlling their bladder or bowels.
- Experience major personality and behavioral changes, including auspiciousness and delusions (such as believing their caregiver is an impostor) or compulsive, repetitive behavior like hand wringing or tissue shredding.

- Tend to wander or become lost.

## Stage 7: Very severe cognitive decline
(Severe or late-stage Alzheimer's)

- In the final stage of this disease, individuals lose the ability to respond to their environment, carry on a conversation and, eventually, to control movement. They may still say words or phrases.

• At this stage, individuals need help with much of their daily personal care, including eating and using the toilet. They may also lose the ability to smile, sit without support and hold their head up. Reflexes become abnormal, muscles grow rigid and swallowing is impaired.

## Symptoms that should be watched out for

Alzheimer's disease (pronounced AHLZ-hi-merz) is one of several disorders that cause the gradual deterioration of brain cells. The disease is named after Dr. Alois Alzheimer, the German physician who first described the disease in 1906.

*The symptoms of Alzheimer's disease include:*

• A gradual loss of memory;

• Problems with learning, reasoning or judgment;

• Loss of language skills;

• Disorientation; and

• A decline in the ability to perform routine tasks.

People with Alzheimer's may also experience changes in their personalities, and exhibit behavioral problems such as agitation, anxiety and delusion.

The progression of Alzheimer's varies significantly and can be difficult to predict. The area of the brain that controls memory and thinking skills is affected first, but, as the disease advances, other regions of the brain and the functions they control may also be affected.

According to the Alzheimer's Association, approximately four million Americans suffer from Alzheimer's. Ageing is the major risk factor for the disease, which strikes men and women in almost equal numbers, and affects almost fifty percent of all people aged eighty-five and older. A family history of the disease also increases one's risk. The most commonly prescribed medications for Alzheimer's disease are a class of drugs known as acetylcholinesterase inhibitors. These are designed to prevent the breakdown of acetylcholine; a chemical messenger in the brain that is important for memory and reasoning.

Some patients who take acetylcholinesterase inhibitors experience a modest, but temporary improvement in cognitive functioning. However, Alzheimer's disease is not yet curable and the available treatment neither halts nor reverses the progression of the illness.

I can't say "**The End**" as it is a new beginning to life!

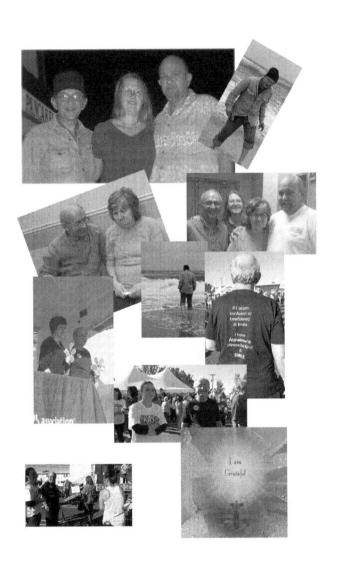

# ABOUT THE AUTHOR

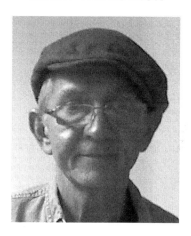

I was born in Manhattan, NY, but most of my life was spent in New Jersey and I traveled the country extensively...and did some overseas travel.

It is the little things in life that matter.

It was very early on in life I started studying human behavior. I guess it was a form of security for me—knowing what every footstep meant, every tone of the voice, and each facial expression or hand gesture. Funny thing, with words I always had problems expressing them, yet give me crayons, and I would draw you a picture, give me a guitar I would play you my music. Basically give me anything and I will create something. There is always some way of expressing myself with this over blown imagination of mine.

There was one moment in my life, however, when I thought I would lose my imagination forever: when I learned that I had Alzheimer's disease.

Despite the diagnosis, I am LUCKY.

I was tested several times... PET scan verified plaque and brain shrinkage! I started taking some natural supplements and with them and the exercising, I have had notable improvement. Math, logic, short-term memory ...all improved and still improving!

I have established a group to help others with Alzheimer's, dementia and memory loss issues.

http://www.endalzmemoryloss.org/
https://www.facebook.com/RobertLRuisi

# Other General Adult Books

*The Panhandler Diaries*

*Hitchhiker*

*The Unknown Stories (anthology)*

*The Three Letters Anthology*

*Dancing into the Fog*

*Sunlight*

*Turning Point*

# Special and Humble Thanks

Susan Grant, M.D. (my angel)
44 Sycamore Avenue, Ste 3-D
Little Silver, New Jersey 07739
732-567-1519

Jersey Shore Neurology Associates, P.A.
Richard Rhee, M.D., PA.
1900 Corlies Avenue
Neptune, New Jersey 07753
732-775-2400

Joel Ross, M.D.
Memory Enhancement Center of America, Inc.
4 Industrial Way West
2nd Floor Eatontown
New Jersey 07724
732-571-1535

Riverview Medical Center
Family Health Center
Dr. Cindy McVey
1 River Plaza
Red Bank, New Jersey 07701

Meridian Health
Riverview Medical Center
For the charity care that they kindly provided

Laura Hawkins
alznj.org
400 Morris Avenue, Suite 251
Denville, NJ 07834
Phone: 973-586-4300

Paul Stamets
Fungi Perfecti LLC
PO Box 7634
Olympia WA 98507
1-800-780-9126
http://www.fungi.com

Jersey Medical Associates, Inc.
Vimutha Raj, M.D.
80 Hazlet Avenue
Hazlet, NJ 07730
732-264-0400

And countless others that have helped me along the way, last but by far not least my 3 daughters and 7 grandchildren that have shown remarkable support over the past few years.

State of New Jersey
PRESCRIPTION BLANK
RIVERVIEW MEDICAL CENTER
FAMILY HEALTH CENTER
1 RIVERVIEW PLAZA, RED BANK, NJ 07701

TEL: (732) 530-2295
FAX: (732) 224-2907
BATCH #

PRINT CLEARLY
CINDY MCKEY NP/A RRETOV

26NN0950400 18119429

PATIENT Ruisi, Robert

11-

Rx
Aricept 5 mg
tab
(#30)
Sig: T tab po

DO NOT REFILL
REFILL

Cindy McKe

---

State of New Jersey
PRESCRIPTION BLANK
RIVERVIEW MEDICAL CENTER
FAMILY HEALTH CENTER
1 RIVERVIEW PLAZA, RED BANK, NJ 07701

TEL: (732) 530-2295
FAX: (732) 224-2907
BATCH # DEA 2022157806

PRINT CLEARLY

2500331258   11/06/12   MDC usu
RUISI ROBERT

Rx
Refer to neurol
n Rhee
dementia

---

State of New Jersey
PRESCRIPTION BLANK
JERSEY SHORE NEUROLOGY ASSOCIATES, P.A.
RICHARD S. RHEE, M.D., F.A.A.N.
NEUROLOGIST
1900 CORLIES AVENUE, NEPTUNE, NJ 07753
TEL: 732-775-2400 • FAX: 732-775-5673
DEA# AR7971597   NPI# 1053046112   LIC# 25MA02610700
SERIAL# 001316
BATCH# NEL14042425046

PATIENT To whom it may
ADDRESS

Rx   Concern   6/3/14

please be advised that
Mr Robert Ruisi suffers from
Alzheimer disease

n Rhee

Made in the USA
Charleston, SC
18 November 2016